100 Questions & Answers About Prostate Cancer

Second Edition

Pamela Ellsworth, MD

Department of Urology
Brown University Medical Center
Providence, Rhode Island

JONES AND BARTLETT PUBLISHERS
Sudbury, Massachusetts
BOSTON   TORONTO   LONDON   SINGAPORE

World Headquarters

Jones and Bartlett Publishers
40 Tall Pine Drive
Sudbury, MA 01776
978-443-5000
info@jbpub.com
www.jbpub.com

Jones and Bartlett Publishers
Canada
6339 Ormindale Way
Mississauga, Ontario L5V 1J2
Canada

Jones and Bartlett Publishers
International
Barb House, Barb Mews
London W6 7PA
United Kingdom

Jones and Bartlett's books and products are available through most bookstores and online booksellers. To contact Jones and Bartlett Publishers directly, call 800-832-0034, fax 978-443-8000, or visit our website, www.jbpub.com.

Substantial discounts on bulk quantities of Jones and Bartlett's publications are available to corporations, professional associations, and other qualified organizations. For details and specific discount information, contact the special sales department at Jones and Bartlett via the above contact information or send an email to specialsales@jbpub.com.

The authors, editor, and publisher have made every effort to provide accurate information. However, they are not responsible for errors, omissions, or for any outcomes related to the use of the contents of this book and take no responsibility for the use of the products and procedures described. Treatments and side effects described in this book may not be applicable to all people; likewise, some people may require a dose or experience a side effect that is not described herein. Drugs and medical devices are discussed that may have limited availability controlled by the Food and Drug Administration (FDA) for use only in a research study or clinical trial. Research, clinical practice, and government regulations often change the accepted standard in this field. When consideration is being given to use of any drug in the clinical setting, the health care provider or reader is responsible for determining FDA status of the drug, reading the package insert, and reviewing prescribing information for the most up-to-date recommendations on dose, precautions, and contraindications, and determining the appropriate usage for the product. This is especially important in the case of drugs that are new or seldom used.

Production Credits

Executive Publisher: Christopher Davis
Custom Projects Editor: Kathy Richardson
Production Director: Amy Rose
Production Editor: Daniel Stone
Senior Marketing Manager: Barb Bartoszek
V.P., Manufacturing and Inventory Control:
  Therese Connell

Composition: Spoke & Wheel/Jason Miranda
Cover Design: Kristin E. Ohlin
Printing and Binding: Malloy, Inc.
Cover Printing: Malloy, Inc.

Cover Credits

Top photo: © Martina Ebel/ShutterStock, Inc.; Bottom left photo: © Yuri Arcurs/ShutterStock, Inc.; Bottom right photo: © Philip Hunton/ShutterStock, Inc.

Library of Congress Cataloging-in-Publication Data
Ellsworth, Pamela.
  100 questions & answers about prostate cancer / Pamela Ellsworth. — 2nd ed.
    p. cm.
  Includes bibliographical references and index.
  ISBN-13: 978-0-7637-5205-7
  ISBN-10: 0-7637-5205-3
  1. Prostate—Cancer—Popular works. 2. Prostate—Cancer—Miscellanea. I. Title. II. Title: 100 questions and answers about prostate cancer. III. Title: One hundred questions and answers about prostate cancer.
  RC280.P7E44 2009
  616.99'463--dc22
                                    2008029341
6048

Printed in the United States of America
14 13 12   10 9 8 7 6 5 4

CONTENTS

If you're reading this book, you're probably concerned about your chances (or a loved one's) of getting prostate cancer—or you may even have been diagnosed with prostate cancer already. Like many people at risk for a disease like prostate cancer, you may wish to be proactive about your health—to read and learn about this disease so you understand how it's diagnosed and treated in order to more effectively make decisions about your health care. And you may be finding out that getting accurate, understandable information about prostate cancer isn't all that easy, despite the multitude of information sources available in the Internet age.

Information on how to screen for, diagnose, and treat prostate cancer comes in many forms, but sometimes it's difficult to follow up on it. When a newspaper article reports promising new treatments being tested at a prominent university hospital, but there's no indication as to whether approval is imminent, how do you learn more? You see on television that the FDA has approved several new drugs for use in prostate cancer; how do you find out about them, and how do you determine which one is best? A Web search of the term "prostate cancer" will bring up hundreds, if not thousands, of web sites with topics ranging from scientific studies of the molecular biology of cancer, to inspirational stories about cancer survivors, to rumors, myths, and wild exaggerations about the causes of prostate cancer. How does anyone—particularly a person who never thought about cancer before and hoped he'd never have to—make sense of all this?

The information in this book is a synthesis of current medical standards, advice based on our experience as both physician and patient, and good, old-fashioned, practical common sense. We wrote this book to help newly diagnosed patients make sense of the diagnosis and learn some of the things you can expect will happen.

Above all, we want readers to understand that you can and should ask questions, request help when you need it, and actively participate in making decisions about your treatment.

The book is divided into seven parts. Part 1 describes the prostate's anatomy and functions and discusses warning signs of prostate disease. Parts 2–4 describe what happens prior to treatment for prostate cancer: the risk factors, screening procedures, diagnosis, and staging of prostate cancer. Part 5 discusses treatment options for prostate cancer, and Part 6 describes treatment of some of the complications that arise with cancer treatment, including bone pain, incontinence, and erectile dysfunction. Part 7 addresses some of the day-to-day problems often faced by prostate cancer patients in coping with their diagnosis, treatment, and complications. An Appendix of resources is included to help readers find additional information.

The question and answer format seemed to be the most sensible way to address some of the most common questions asked by real patients. Naturally, we could not include all possible questions about prostate cancer, nor could we cover all topics as thoroughly as we would like. Thus, we've tried to present the best information available on many important topics while pointing our readers in the direction of high-quality sources of information and encouraging them to ask questions and seek assistance from their own physicians. We hope that our efforts will help some of the many men (and their families) who will confront prostate cancer in the months and years to come.

This book is dedicated to the men with prostate cancer, along with their families, with whom I have had the opportunity to work during the evaluation, treatment, and follow-up of their cancer throughout my residency and postresidency years. It is also dedicated to those gentlemen that I follow for prostate cancer screening. These individuals have allowed me to capture a glimpse of the magnitude of this disease and its effect on the individual and his family. All too often, we surgeons and physicians lose sight of the individual and the family in our attempts to "eradicate disease." Yet the prevalence of prostate cancer, the controversy over screening, the variety of treatment options, and the potential for treatment options to adversely affect quality of life bring to light the need for an individual-centered approach to the treatment of prostate cancer. Choosing from the variety of treatment options, each with unique benefits and risks, as well as the "watchful waiting" approach may prove overwhelming in this era of patient-driven decision making. As physicians, it is our job to educate our patients and their spouses or significant others so that they may make the most appropriate decision. Those who have shared their anger, sorrow, frustration, enthusiasm, and joy during the process of diagnosis, treatment, and follow-up have underscored the need for such extensive and personal communication. It is my hope that this book will help individuals diagnosed with or concerned about prostate cancer with some of the questions that they, their spouse, or significant others may have. I also hope that it will stimulate them to ask such questions of their physician, no matter how trivial they may perceive these questions to be.

Since writing the first edition of this book there have been several important changes in the evaluation and management of prostate cancer. The *Second Edition* has been written to keep patients and their families aware of the changes that are occuring in this area of urology. This edition will address such important changes as the advent of robotic prostatectomy. New screening tests for the detection of prostate cancer that are currently under investigation are also reviewed. Medications that are used to treat prostate cancer and the side effects of prostate cancer treatment have been updated.

I would like to thank Dr. Steven Rous for giving me the opportunity to find out how rewarding writing can be and for being a true mentor. A special thanks goes to Oliver Gill for his willingness to write about his personal experiences. Lastly, thanks to Jones and Bartlett Publishers for their willingness to print a second edition so that patients and their families can remain "up to date" in terms of the evaluation and management of prostate cancer.

Pamela Ellsworth, MD

PART ONE

The Basics

What is the prostate gland and what does it do?

Do women have a prostate gland and PSA?

What are the signs and symptoms of an enlarged
prostate (either cancer-related or benign)?

More . . .

1. What is the prostate gland and what does it do?

The prostate gland is actually not a single gland; rather, it is composed of a collection of glands that are covered by a capsule. A **gland** is a structure or organ that produces a substance that is used in another part of the body. The prostate gland lies below the bladder, encircles the **urethra** (the tube through which one urinates), and lies in front of the rectum. Because it lies just in front of the rectum, the **posterior** (back) aspect of the prostate can be assessed during a rectal examination. The normal size of the prostate gland is about the size of a walnut (**Figures 1** and **2**).

Gland

A structure or organ that produces substances that affect other areas of the body.

Urethra

The tube that runs from the bladder neck to the tip of the penis through which urine passes.

Posterior

The rear or back side.

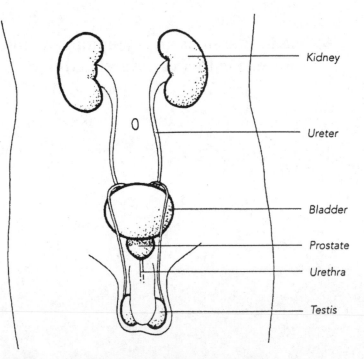

0

Kidney

Ureter

Bladder

Prostate

Urethra

Testis

Figure 1 Anatomy of the male genitourinary system.
From *Prostate and Cancer* by Sheldon H. F. Marks. Copyright © 1995 by Sheldon Marks. Reprinted by permission of Perseus Books Publishers, a member of Perseus Books, LLC.

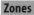
The prostate gland is divided into several **zones**, or areas. These divisions are based on locations of the tissue, but they also have some significance with respect to prostate cancer. The different zones are the transition zone, the peripheral zone, and the central zone (**Figure 3**). In most prostate cancers, the tumor occurs in the peripheral zone. In a few cases, the tumor is mostly located in the transition zone, around the urethra or toward the abdomen. In 85% of cases, the prostate cancer is **multifocal**, meaning that it is found in more than one area in the prostate. Seventy percent of prostate cancer patients with a **palpable nodule**, one that can be felt by a rectal examination, have cancer on the other side also. Another way to describe the prostate gland is to divide it into lobes. The prostate gland has five lobes: two lateral lobes, a middle lobe, an anterior lobe, and a posterior lobe. **Benign** (noncancerous) enlargement of the prostate typically occurs in the lateral lobes and may also affect the middle lobe.

Zones

An area of the prostate distinguished from adjacent areas.

Multifocal

Found in more than one area.

Palpable

Capable of being felt during a physical examination by an experienced doctor. In the case of prostate cancer, this refers to an abnormality of the prostate that can be felt during a rectal examination.

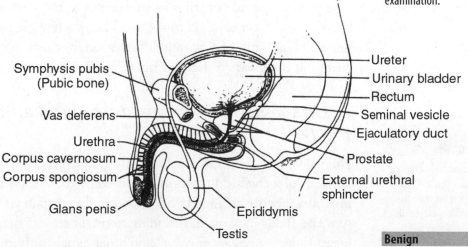

Figure 2 Anatomy of the male genitourinary system.

Rous, Stephen. *The Prostate Book Sound Advice on Symptoms and Treatment*, Copyright © 1994, W. W. Norton & Co.

Benign

A growth that is not cancerous.

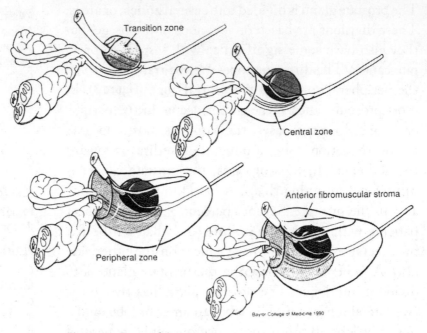

Figure 3 Zones of the prostate.
Reprinted with permission from McNeal JE: Normal Histology of the Prostate. *Am J Surg Pathol* 1988; 12(8): 619–633.

The prostate gland contributes substances to the ejaculate that serve as nutrients to sperm. The prostate gland has a high amount of zinc in it. The reason for this is not clear, but it appears to help in fighting off infections.

2. Do women have a prostate gland and PSA?

Prostate specific antigen (PSA)

A chemical produced by benign and cancerous prostate tissue. The level tends to be higher with prostate cancer.

No, women do not have prostate glands. However, small amounts of a chemical typically produced by the prostate, **prostate-specific antigen (PSA)**, are found in certain tissues and fluids in women, including normal breast tissue, breast fluid, breast cancer tissue, and other female tumors.

3. What are the signs and symptoms of an enlarged prostate (either cancer-related or benign)?

The prostate gland in the adult male is normally about 20 to 25 cm^3 in size. Over time, the prostate gland may grow as a result of benign enlargement of the prostate, known as **benign prostatic hyperplasia (BPH),** or as a result of prostate cancer. Enlargement of the prostate gland may cause changes in urinary symptoms; however, the severity of urinary symptoms does not correlate with the size of the prostate. In fact, some men with mildly enlarged prostates (for example, 40 cm^3) may be more symptomatic than men with greatly enlarged (> 100 cm^3) prostate glands. The symptoms of an enlarged prostate are caused by the prostate's resistance to the outflow of urine and the bladder's response to this resistance. Common symptoms include

- Getting up at night to urinate more often than one time per night (**nocturia**)
- Urinating more frequently than every two hours during the daytime
- Feeling that you have to urinate, but when you attempt to, finding that it takes a while for the urine to come out (**hesitancy**)
- Straining or pushing to get your urine stream started and/or to maintain your stream
- Dribbling urine near the completion of voiding
- A urine stream that stops and starts during voiding (**intermittency**)
- Feeling of incomplete emptying after voiding such that you feel that you could void again shortly

THE BASICS

BPH (benign prostatic hyperplasia)
Noncancerous enlargement of the prostate.

Nocturia
Awakening at night with the desire to void.

Hesitancy
A delay in the start of the urine stream during voiding.

Intermittency
An inability to complete voiding and empty the bladder with one single contraction of the bladder. A stopping and starting of the urine stream during urination.

4. What is PSA? What is the normal PSA value?

PSA stands for prostate specific antigen. PSA is a chemical that is produced by prostate cells, both normal and cancerous. PSA is not produced significantly by other cells in the body. Normally, only a small amount of PSA gets into the bloodstream. However, when the prostate is irritated, inflamed, or damaged, such as in prostatitis and prostate cancer, PSA leaks into the bloodstream more easily, causing the level of PSA in the blood to be higher. The normal range is usually 0 to 4 ng/mL; however, in younger men a lower range is used (**Table 1**). The normal range for PSA varies with age and race.

Once a baseline normal PSA has been obtained, the actual number becomes less important and the rate of change of the PSA over time becomes more important.

5. What is free : total PSA?

PSA is found in two forms in the bloodstream: PSA that is attached to chemicals (proteins) is **bound PSA**, and PSA that is not attached to proteins is called **free PSA**. The amount of each form is measured, and a ratio of the free PSA to the free plus bound (or total) PSA is calculated.

Bound PSA

PSA attached to the proteins in the bloodstream.

Free PSA

The PSA present that is not bound to proteins. It is often expressed as a ratio of free PSA to total PSA in terms of percent, which is the free PSA divided by the total PSA × 100.

Table 1 Age-Adjusted Normal PSA Ranges

Age (yr)	Normal range (ng/mL)
40–49	0–2.5 (0–2.0 for African Americans)
50–59	0–3.5
60–69	0–4.5
70–79	0–6.5

Reprinted with permission from Oesterling et al, *JAMA* 1993;270:860–864. Copyright © American Medical Association.

The higher this number, the less likely that prostate cancer is present. A free PSA value greater than 14–25% suggests that the presence of prostate cancer is less likely. This ratio may be helpful in individuals with mildly elevated PSAs in the 4–10 ng/mL range for whom the doctor is deciding whether to perform a prostate biopsy.

6. What causes the PSA to rise?

Anything that irritates or inflames the prostate can increase the PSA, such as a urinary tract infection, prostate stones, a recent urinary catheter or cystoscopy (a look into the bladder through a specialized telescope-like instrument), recent prostate biopsy, or prostate surgery. Sexual intercourse may increase the PSA up to 10%, and a vigorous rectal examination or prostatic massage before the PSA blood test is drawn may also increase the PSA. Benign enlargement of the prostate (BPH) may also increase the PSA because more prostate cells are present, thus more PSA is produced. Benign prostatic hyperplasia tends to produce less PSA than prostate cancer, so with BPH the PSA density (the amount of PSA/volume of prostate) is lower than with prostate cancer. Because the prostate gland can continue to grow as one ages, the PSA may increase slightly from year to year, reflecting this growth. Some argue that the PSA should not change by more than 0.7 ng/mL per year or by 20% of the previous level if the increase is secondary to benign growth of the prostate. The rate of change in the PSA over a period of time is called the **PSA velocity**.

PSA velocity

The rate of change of the PSA over a period of time (change in PSA/change in time).

7. Are there medications that may affect the PSA? Does testosterone therapy cause the PSA to increase?

Yes, some medications can affect the PSA. Five (5) alpha-reductase inhibitors are a class of medication used to shrink the prostate in men with benign enlargement of the prostate, decreasing the PSA by 50%. This decrease in PSA occurs predictably no matter what your initial PSA is. Any sustained increases in PSA while you are on a 5-alpha-reductase inhibitor (provided you are taking it regularly) should be evaluated. The percentage of free PSA (the amount of free PSA divided by the amount of total PSA) is not significantly decreased by these medications and should remain stable while you are on them. Medications can decrease the amount of testosterone produced by your testicles and may decrease the PSA. Decreasing the amount of testosterone may cause both benign and cancerous prostate tissue to shrink. Testosterone is broken down in the body to a chemical, dihydrotestosterone, which is responsible for the stimulation of prostate growth. Thus, the addition of testosterone may stimulate the growth of normal prostate cells and possibly prostate cancer cells. Because normal prostate cells produce PSA, it is not unreasonable to expect that an increase in the normal cells present in the prostate would lead to an increase in the PSA. Prostate cancer is composed of both hormone-sensitive and hormone-insensitive cells. The hormone-insensitive cells grow regardless of the availability of testosterone or its breakdown products, whereas the hormone-sensitive cells appear to be dependent on the male hormone for growth. Thus, the addition of testosterone may affect the growth of these hormone-sensitive cells. Testosterone therapy has not been shown to cause the development of prostate cancer.

8. Is there anything special that I should do if I am on testosterone therapy?

Because there is theoretical risk that testosterone therapy can cause an undetected prostate cancer to grow, you should have a digital rectal examination and get a PSA level every six months rather than yearly. If there is a significant increase in your PSA or a change in your rectal examination while you are on testosterone therapy, the testosterone should be discontinued and a transrectal ultrasound (TRUS)–guided prostate biopsy should be performed.

9. Can I have my PSA done anywhere?

It is best to have your PSA obtained at the same lab each time because different labs may use different forms of PSA testing. The PSA Hybritech Tandem-R PSA test can detect PSA at a level of 0.1 ng/mL, whereas some of the newer PSA tests, such as the Abbott IMx, Yang Proscheck, and Diagnostic Products Immulite, can detect PSA at levels of 0.01–0.04 ng/mL. To minimize lab variability and to avoid unnecessary anxiety, repeat blood tests, or biopsy, it is best to have your PSA performed by the same lab each year.

10. Are there any other markers for prostate cancer?

Early Prostate Cancer Antigen (EPCA) and EPCA-2 have been demonstrated to be plasma-based markers for prostate cancer. EPCA is found throughout the prostate and represents a "field effect" associated with prostate cancer, whereas, EPCA-2 is found only in the prostate cancer tissue, but is able to get into the plasma, the liquid part of the blood, allowing for it to be detected by a blood test. In preliminary studies, EPCA-2 has been able to identify men with prostate cancer who had normal PSA levels (> 2.5 ng/ml). This data, however, is preliminary and further studies are needed to validate the sensitivity and specificity of these markers.

PART TWO

Prostate Cancer

What is prostate cancer?

How common is prostate cancer?

What are the risk factors for prostate cancer, and who is at risk? Is there anything that decreases the risk of developing prostate cancer?

More . . .

11. What is prostate cancer?

Cell

The smallest unit of the body. Tissues in the body are made up of cells.

Tumor

Abnormal tissue growth that may be cancerous or noncancerous (benign).

Cancer

Abnormal and uncontrolled growth of cells in the body that may spread, injure areas of the body, and lead to death.

Malignancy

Uncontrolled growth of cells that can spread to other areas of the body and cause death.

Lymph

A clear fluid that is found throughout the body. Lymph fluid helps fight infections.

Lymph node(s)

Small bean-shaped glands that are found throughout the body. Lymph fluid passes through the lymph nodes, which filter out bacteria, cancer cells, and toxic chemicals.

Prostate cancer is a malignant growth of the glandular cells of the prostate. Our body is composed of billions of **cells**; they are the smallest unit in the body. Normally, each cell functions for a while, then dies and is replaced in an organized manner. This results in the appropriate number of cells being present to carry out necessary cell functions. Sometimes there can be an uncontrolled replacement of cells, leaving the cells unable to organize as they did before. Such abnormal growth of cells is called a **tumor**. Tumors may be benign (noncancerous) or malignant (cancerous). **Cancer** is abnormal cell growth and disorder such that the "cancer cells" can grow without the normal controls and limits. A **malignancy** is a cancerous growth that has the potential to spread and cause damage to other tissues of the body or even lead to death. Cancers can spread locally into surrounding tissues, or cancer cells can break away from the tumor and enter body fluids, such as the blood and lymph, and spread to other parts of the body. **Lymph** is an almost-clear fluid that drains waste from cells. This fluid travels in vessels to the **lymph nodes**, small bean-shaped structures that filter unwanted substances, such as cancer cells and bacteria, out of the fluid. Lymph nodes may become filled with cancer cells.

As with most cancers, prostate cancer is not contagious.

12. How common is prostate cancer?

There are more than 100 different types of cancer. In the United States, a man has a 50% chance of developing some type of cancer in his lifetime. In American men, (excluding skin cancer) prostate cancer is the most common cancer. Prostate cancer accounts for about 33%

(234,460) cases of cancer (**Table 2**). More than 75% of the cases of prostate cancer are diagnosed in men older than 65. Based on cases diagnosed between 1995 and 2001, it is estimated that 91% of the new cases of prostate cancer are expected to be diagnosed at local or regional stages (see staging of prostate cancer, chapter 3, question 27) for which 5-year survival is nearly 100%. It is estimated that prostate cancer will be the cause of death in 9% of men, 27,350 prostate-cancer related deaths. In the United States, deaths from prostate cancer have decreased significantly by 4.1% per year from 1994 to 2004. Most notably, the death rate for African-American men in the United States has decreased by 6%.

13. What are the risk factors for prostate cancer, and who is at risk? Is there anything that decreases the risk of developing prostate cancer?

Theoretically, all men are at risk for developing prostate cancer. The prevalence of prostate cancer increases with age, and the increase with age is greater for prostate cancer than for any other cancer.

Table 2 Cancer Statistics for Men in the United States—2009

Cancer Site	Estimated % of All New Cancer Diagnoses	Estimated Number of New Cases
Prostate	25%	192,280
Digestive system	10%	75,590
Lung and bronchus	15%	116,090

Reprinted with permission from Jemal A, Siegel R, Ward E, Hao Y, Xu J, Thun MJ. *Cancer Statistics*, 2009. CA Cancer J Clin 2009 Jul-Aug; 59(4): 225-49.

1:10,000   < 39 years of age

1:103   40–59 years of age

1:8   60–79 years of age

Basically, every ten years after the age of 40, the incidence of prostate cancer nearly doubles, with a risk of 10% for men in their 50s increasing to 70% for those in their 80s. However, in most older men, the prostate cancer does not grow; many die of other causes and are not identified as having prostate cancer before their death.

Prostate cancer is 66% more common among African-Americans, and it is twice as likely to be fatal in African-Americans as in Caucasians. However, blacks in Africa have one of the lowest rates of prostate cancer in the world. Males of Asian descent living in the United States have lower rates of prostate cancer than Caucasians, but higher rates than Asian males in their native countries. Japan appears to have the lowest prostate cancer death rate, compared with Switzerland, which has the highest (**Figure 4**).

Castration

The removal of both testicles.

Prostate cancer is related to sex hormones. Prostate cancer rarely develops in men who had their testicles removed (**castration**) at an early age. There is a correlation between prostate cancer and high levels of testosterone. There does not appear to be any clear correlation between body size and risk of prostate cancer; however, men with prostate cancer who had weight gain in early adulthood tend to have more aggressive cancers. Smoking does not appear to increase your risk of cancer; however, smokers tend to have more aggressive cancer than nonsmokers. Physical activity appears to decrease the risk of prostate cancer.

The effects of vasectomy on the risk of prostate cancer are unclear. Some studies have demonstrated an increased

PROSTATE CANCER

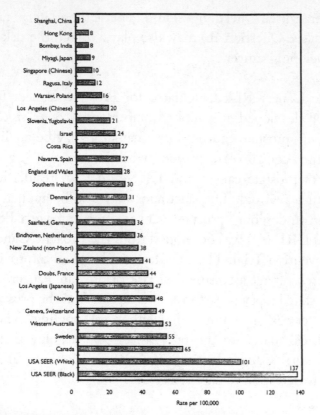

Figure 4 International prostate cancer incidence rates—1998.
Stanford JL, Stephenson RA, Coyle LM et al. Prostate Cancer Trends 1973-1995. Bethesda MD.
Cancer Surveillance, Epidemiology, and End Results (SEER) Program, National Cancer Institute 1998.

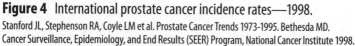

risk of prostate cancer with vasectomy, but these individuals tended to have a lower-grade, lower-stage prostate cancer that is associated with a better prognosis. Other studies have failed to confirm an increased risk of prostate cancer after vasectomy. **Vasectomy** is the minor surgical sterilization procedure in which the **vas deferens** (the sperm duct) is cut and either clipped, tied, or cauterized to prevent it from reattaching itself. Vasectomy does not affect testosterone production or release of testosterone from the testicles into the bloodstream; it only prevents sperm from leaving the testis. Current medical wisdom holds that vasectomy does not increase your risk of prostate cancer.

Vasectomy

A procedure in which the vas deferens are cut and tied off, clipped, or cauterized to prevent the exit of sperm from the testicles. It makes a man sterile.

Vas deferens

A tiny tube that connects the testicles to the urethra through which sperm passes.

Dietary (see Question 17) and genetic (hereditary) factors (see Question 16) may also play a role in the risk of developing cancer.

The Cancer Risk Calculator for Prostate Cancer has been developed as a tool to help identify one's risk of having prostate cancer. The calculator may be applied to men age 50 years or older, with no previous diagnosis of prostate cancer and DRE and PSA results less than 1 year old. The calculator may also be applied to men undergoing prostate cancer screening with PSA and DRE as it was developed from the Prostate Cancer Prevention Trial. The calculator is designed to provide a preliminary assessment of risk of prostate cancer if a prostate biopsy is performed. One can find the prostate cancer risk calculator online, either by Googling "cancer risk calculator for prostate cancer" or by going to the National Cancer Institute website and looking under early detection research network.

14. I have a family member with prostate cancer. Am I at risk?

In certain cases, it appears that the risk for prostate cancer is passed on to males in the family. The younger the family member is when he is diagnosed with prostate cancer, the higher the risk is for male relatives to have prostate cancer at a younger age. The risk also increases with the number of relatives affected with prostate cancer (**Table 3**).

15. I have sons. Are they at risk for prostate cancer and, if so, at what age should they start screening?

Yes, there is an increased risk for all male relatives, including brothers, sons, cousins, and nephews. Your sons' risk varies with your age at detection. The younger you are at diagnosis, the higher the risk for your sons. If your age is 72 or older at the time of diagnosis of prostate cancer, then your sons' risk is probably no greater than that of the general population.

Table 3 Relative Risk for Prostate Cancer with Affected Relatives

Age of Onset (Years)	Additional Relatives Beyond One First-Degree Relative Affected	Relative Risk
70	None	1.0
60	None	1.4
50	None	2.0
70	One or more	4.0
60	One or more	5.0
50	One or more	7.0

Reprinted with permission from Carter BS, Bovea GS, Beaty TH et al. J Urol 1993;150:797–802.

Screening of your sons should begin at age 40, and a digital rectal examination should be performed and a PSA obtained, both of which should be repeated yearly thereafter.

Screening of your sons should begin at age 40, and a digital rectal examination should be performed and a PSA obtained, both of which should be repeated yearly thereafter. It may also be helpful for your sons to make some preventive dietary and lifestyle changes now (see Question 17).

16. Are there genes that put people at risk for prostate cancer?

It is thought that 9% of all prostate cancers, and more than 40% of prostate cancers occurring in younger males, are related to genetic causes. Abnormalities of genes of chromosomes I and the X chromosome are associated with an increased risk of prostate cancer. One such gene, the HPC1 gene, appears to cause about one third of all inherited cases of prostate cancer. There also appears to be a gene that is carried on the X chromosome (the chromosome passed on to the male by his mother) that may increase the risk of prostate cancer. This X chromosome-related increased risk of prostate cancer might somehow play a part in the identification of a higher incidence of prostate cancer in male relatives of women with breast cancer.

17. How does my diet affect my risk of prostate cancer?

A variety of dietary risk factors exist for prostate cancer. Several studies suggest that a high-fat diet stimulates prostate cancer to grow; in particular, beef and high-fat dairy products appear to be stimulators of prostate cancer. Conversely, a low-fat diet rich in fruits and vegetables may help decrease the risk of prostate cancer.

Such "healthy" foods include soy (tofu and soy milk), tomatoes, green tea, red grapes, strawberries, raspberries, blueberries, peas, watermelon, rosemary, garlic, and citrus. Soy contains substances called phytoestrogens, which resemble the female sex hormone estrogen. In dietary doses—that is, amounts normally found in foods, not the amounts in supplements—phytoestrogens can decrease the risk of prostate cancer. Green tea contains **antioxidants**, which are chemicals that may help prevent cellular damage.

Antioxidant

A chemical that may help prevent cellular damage.

Vitamin E is a free-radical scavenger and is also associated with a decreased risk of prostate cancer, but men with a history of bleeding problems or who take blood thinners should discuss the use of vitamin E with their doctor before taking it.

A high intake of dairy products has also been associated with an increased risk of prostate cancer.

Vitamin D deficiency has been associated with an increased risk of prostate cancer.

High levels of fructose, a form of sugar, have been associated with a lower risk of prostate cancer. Selenium has been associated with a decreased risk of prostate cancer. Lycopene, a carotenoid (chemicals that give orange, red, or yellow coloring to plants), is associated with a decreased risk of prostate cancer. Lycopene is found in high levels in tomatoes and is beneficial only if one eats cooked tomatoes, such as tomato sauce, not tomato juice. Many studies are in the process of looking at the effects of such dietary risks.

18. Do African Americans have a higher risk of prostate cancer?

Black men are more likely to get prostate cancer at a younger age, and they often have a more aggressive cancer.

Black men are more likely to get prostate cancer at a younger age, and they often have a more aggressive cancer. Of all population groups in the world, African-American men have the highest rate of prostate cancer. The reason for this is not known. Because they are at higher risk, African-American men should start prostate cancer screening at a younger age than Caucasian men (see Question 28).

19. What are the warning signs of prostate cancer?

Prostate cancer gives no typical warning signs that it is present in your body. It often grows very slowly, and some of the symptoms related to enlargement of the prostate are typical of noncancerous enlargement of the prostate, known as benign prostatic hyperplasia (BPH).

With more advanced disease, you may have fatigue, weight loss, and generalized aches and pains.

When the disease has spread to the bones, it may cause pain in the area. Bone pain may present in different ways. In some men, it may cause continuous pain, while in others, the pain may be intermittent. It may be confined to a particular area of the body or move around the body; it may be variable during the day and respond differently to rest and activity. If there is significant weakening of the bone(s), fractures (breaks in the bone) may occur. More common sites of bone metastases include the hips, back, ribs, and shoulders. Some of these sites are also common locations for arthritis, so the presence of pain in any of these areas is not definitive for prostate cancer.

If prostate cancer spreads locally to the lymph nodes, it often does not cause any symptoms. Rarely, if there is extensive lymph node involvement, leg swelling may occur.

In patients with advanced cancer that has spread to the spine, paralysis can occur if the nerves are compressed because of either collapse of the spine or tumor growing into the spine.

If the prostate cancer grows into the floor (bottom) of the bladder, or if a large amount of cancer is present in the pelvic lymph nodes, one or both ureters (the tubes that drain urine from the kidneys into the bladder) can be obstructed. Signs and symptoms of ureteral obstruction include decreased urine volume, no urine volume if both **ureters** are blocked, back pain, nausea, vomiting, and possibly fevers if infections occur.

Blood in the urine and blood in the ejaculate are usually not related to prostate cancer; however, if these are present, you should seek urologic evaluation.

In individuals with widespread metastatic disease, bleeding problems can occur. In addition, patients with prostate cancer may develop anemia. The anemia may be related to extensive tumor in the bone, hormonal therapy, or the length of time you have had the cancer. Because the blood count tends to drop slowly, you may not have any symptoms of anemia. Some individuals with very significant anemia may have weakness, orthostatic hypotension (lowering of the blood pressure when you stand up), dizziness, shortness of breath, and the feeling of being ill and tired. Symptoms of advanced disease and their treatments are listed in **Table 4**.

Ureters

Tubes that connect the kidneys to the bladder, through which urine passes into the bladder.

Table 4 Common Symptom-Directed Treatment Strategies in Advanced Prostate Cancer

Symptom	Treatment

Bone pain	• Irradiation
	  – Localized metastasis: external beam
	  – Widespread metastasis: total body irradiation;
	    intravenous infusion
	• Bisphosphonates
	• Steroids
	• Chemotherapy
	• Analgesics
	  – NSAIDs
	  – Narcotic agents

Bone fracture	• Surgical stabilization
Bladder obstruction	• Hormonal treatment • Transurethral prostatectomy • Repeated debulking transurethral resections • Alum irrigation • Urethral catheter balloon intervention ($\leq$ 24 hr) • Surgery
Ureteral obstruction	• Endocrine therapy • Radiation therapy • Percutaneous nephrostomy • Indwelling ureteral stents
Spinal cord compression	• Intravenous and/or oral steroids • Posterior laminectomy • Radiation therapy
Dissemination intravascular coagulation (DIC)	• Intravenous herparin and EACA • Supplementation (e.g., platelets, fresh whole blood, packed • erythrocytes, frozen plasma, or cryoprecipitate)
Anemia	• Iron and vitamin supplementation • Bone marrow stimulants • Transfusion therapy
Edema	• Compression stockings • Leg elevation • Diuretics

EACA = epsilon aminocaproic acid; NSAIDs = nonsteroidal anti-inflammatory drugs. From Smith JA et al., *Urology* 1999; 54 (suppl 6A):8–14. Reprinted with permission from Elsevier Science.

20. What causes prostate cancer?

The exact causes of prostate cancer are not known. Prostate cancer may develop because of changes in genes. Alterations in androgen (male hormone) related genes have been associated with an increased risk of cancer. Alterations in genes may be caused by environmental factors, such as diet. The more abnormal the gene, the higher is the likelihood of developing prostate cancer. In rare cases, prostate cancer may be inherited. In such cases, 88% of the individuals will have prostate cancer by the age of 85 years. Males who have a particular gene, the breast cancer mutation (BRCA1), have a threefold higher risk of developing prostate cancer than do other men. Changes in a certain chromosome, p53, in prostate cancer are associated with high-grade aggressive prostate cancer.

21. What causes prostate cancer to grow?

Prostate cancer, similar to breast cancer, is hormone sensitive. Prostate cancer growth is stimulated by the male hormones testosterone and dihydrotestosterone (a chemical that the body makes from testosterone). Testosterone is responsible for many normal changes, both physical and behavioral, that occur in a man's life, such as voice change and hair growth. The testis makes almost 90% of the testosterone in the body. A small amount of testosterone is made by the **adrenal glands** (a paired set of glands found above the kidneys that produce a variety of substances and hormones that are essential for daily living). In the bones, a chemical called transferrin, which is made by the liver and stored in the bones, also appears to stimulate the growth of prostate cancer cells. When cancers develop, they secrete chemicals that cause blood vessels to grow into the cancer and bring nutrients to the cancer so that it can grow.

Adrenal glands

Glands located above each kidney. These glands produce several different hormones including sex hormones.

22. Where does prostate cancer spread?

As the prostate cancer grows, it grows through the prostate, the prostate capsule, and the fat that surrounds the prostate capsule. Because the prostate gland lies below the bladder and attaches to it, the prostate cancer can also grow up into the base of the bladder.

Seminal vesicles

Glandular structures that are located above and behind the prostate. They produce fluid that is part of the ejaculate.

Prostate cancer can also grow into the **seminal vesicles** (paired structures that produce fluid that is part of the ejaculate volume), which are located adjacent to the prostate. It may continue to grow locally in the pelvis into muscles within the pelvis; into the rectum, which lies behind the prostate; or into the sidewall of the pelvis. The spread of cancer to other sites is called metastasis. When prostate cancer spreads outside of the capsule and the fatty tissue, it usually goes to two main areas in the body: the lymph nodes that drain the prostate and the bones. The more commonly involved lymph nodes are those in the pelvis (**Figure 5**), and bones that are more commonly affected are the spine (backbones) and the ribs. Less commonly, prostate cancer can spread to solid organs in the body, such as the liver.

**TURP
(transurethral
prostatectomy)**

A surgical technique performed under anesthesia using a specialized instrument similar to the cystoscope that allows the surgeon to remove the prostatic tissue that is bulging into the urethra and blocking the flow of urine through the urethra. After a TURP, the outer rim of the prostate remains.

23. Does having a prior transurethral prostatectomy without detection of any cancer protect or assure me that I don't have and won't develop prostate cancer?

The answer to this question is no for several reasons. Remember, prostate cancer tends to develop in the peripheral zone of the prostate, whereas benign growth of the prostate (BPH) tends to occur in the transition zone. The goal of the **transurethral prostatectomy (TURP)** is to

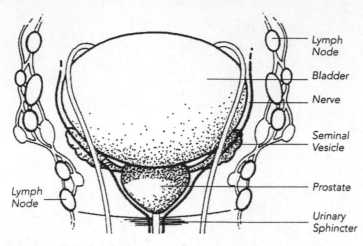

Lymph
Node

Bladder

Nerve

Seminal
Vesicle

Prostate

Urinary
Sphincter

Lymph
Node

Figure 5 Lymph node drainage from the prostate.
From *Prostate and Cancer* by Sheldon H. F. Marks. Copyright © 1995 by Sheldon Marks.
Reprinted by permission of Perseus Books Publishers, a member of Perseus Books, LLC.

remove all of the obstructing prostatic tissue; thus, the
transition zone tissue is resected, and depending on the
skill and thoroughness of your urologist, variable amounts
of the peripheral zone tissue are also resected. However,
TURP does not remove all of your prostate tissue. At
the completion of a TURP, you are still left with the
remaining prostate tissue and thus need to continue with
prostate cancer screening. The only surgical procedure
that removes all prostate tissue is a radical prostatectomy.
Some men with very large prostates undergo an open
prostatectomy for benign enlargement of the prostate.
This procedure does not remove all of the prostate tissue
either; however, it tends to remove more than a TURP.

Remember that you are not born with prostate cancer.
Prostate cancer develops over time, and the incidence
increases with age. Thus, if you had your TURP at a
younger age, there is still a chance that as you age, a prostate cancer will develop, and you should participate in
prostate cancer screening if this is appropriate for you.

PART THREE

Evaluation for Prostate Cancer

How do you detect prostate cancer?

What is prostate cancer screening?

Will my insurance cover prostate cancer screening and treatment?

More . . .

24. How do you detect prostate cancer?

Prostate cancer often does not cause any signs or symptoms, and there are no signs or symptoms specific to prostate cancer. In the earlier stages, it may not cause any perceptible changes in your overall health that will make you aware of the cancer's presence. Currently, a high PSA is the most common indication for prostate biopsy. However, prostate cancer may occur in men with a normal PSA, and this is why the rectal examination is important. Even if you have a normal PSA, you should undergo a prostate biopsy if rectal examination reveals a firm or nodular area. A combination of PSA and a digital rectal examination is the best screening for prostate cancer. Occasionally, prostate cancer is detected when the pathologist examines prostate tissue that was removed during a TURP or open prostatectomy for BPH. This occurs in about 10–15% of individuals with prostate cancer. If prostate cancer is not detected early and is identified in the later stages, it may be detected as part of a work-up for bone pain, urinary tract obstruction, weight loss, or hematuria.

A combination of PSA and a digital rectal examination is the best screening for prostate cancer.

25. What is prostate cancer screening?

The goal of any "screening" is to evaluate populations of people in an effort to diagnose the disease early. Thus, the goal of prostate cancer screening is the early detection of prostate cancer, ideally at the "curable" stage. Prostate cancer screening includes both a digital rectal examination and a serum PSA. Each of these is important in the screening process, and an abnormality in either warrants further evaluation. Only about 25% (one quarter) of prostate cancers are revealed by rectal examination; most are detected by an abnormal PSA. Some studies suggest that even with PSA-based prostate cancer screening, up to 15% of men will have undetected prostate cancer. Newer screening tools, such as EPCA and EPCA-2, are being investigated (see Question 10).

Prostate cancer screening should be performed on a yearly basis, except for men with a very low initial PSA level who may want to consider screening on an every-other-year basis. As you continue with screening on a yearly basis, changes in the PSA (beyond what is believed to be a change caused by benign growth of the prostate) or rectal examination will prompt further evaluation. It is hoped that through the use of prostate cancer screening, the morbidity and mortality associated with prostate cancer will be diminished. More recent studies are showing increased survival as a result of prostate cancer screening.

26. Will my insurance cover prostate cancer screening and treatment?

At this point, Medicare covers annual digital rectal examination and PSA for qualified Medicare patients aged 50 and older. Most health insurance providers are also providing similar coverage. The costs of the various treatments for prostate cancer vary from institution to institution. Most HMOs cover treatment of prostate cancer if the treatment is performed by an HMO-affiliated physician. If you receive care outside of the HMO system, then you may be responsible for the cost of your treatment. If you have questions regarding insurance coverage, it is always best to check with your insurance company before you start screening and treatment to make sure that you are fully aware of your coverage and its possible limitations.

27. Why do some primary care providers discourage or not discuss prostate cancer screening?

The PSA test is a sensitive, but not specific, test for prostate cancer, but elevated PSA can stem from circumstances other than cancer, as noted in Questions 6 and 7. This means that a fair number of men who undergo TRUS-guided prostate biopsies for an elevated PSA do not have prostate cancer, and their worries about cancer are unnecessary. In addition, many argue that with PSA testing, we may be detecting a large number of "clinically **occult**" prostate cancers (cancers that would have gone undetected if not for the PSA test) that would not have caused the individual any harm. Identification and subsequent treatment of such cancers may place the individual at unnecessary risk for erectile dysfunction and voiding troubles. Indeed, detection of occult, non-life-threatening cancers was believed to be the reason for the large number of prostate cancers detected when PSA testing was first used; however, the numbers have decreased, suggesting that this is not entirely the case. Until recently, it was argued that early detection of prostate cancer did not affect survival; however, recent long-term studies have shown a positive impact of prostate cancer screening on prostate cancer-related survival. Currently, no other blood tests or radiographic studies are superior to the combination of digital rectal examination and PSA in the screening for prostate cancer, nor are there any studies that can predict who would get into trouble if his prostate cancer went undetected and untreated.

Prostate cancer screening is not mandatory; it is your choice whether to have prostate cancer screening. You should discuss the pros and cons of prostate cancer

Occult cancer

Cancer that is not detectable through standard physical exams; symptom-free disease.

screening with your primary care provider and consider how it relates to your overall medical health as you make your decision. If you wish to have a PSA test and your primary care provider has not been obtaining PSA levels, then ask for a PSA test. Most insurance companies pay for prostate cancer screening. If yours doesn't, contact your local hospital or urologist's office to get the locations of free testing during Prostate Cancer Awareness Week (see Question 93).

28. When should I start worrying about prostate cancer?

The American Urologic Association (AUA) advises that PSA testing should be offered to well-informed men age 40 years or older who have a life expectancy of at least 10 years.

29. When should one stop having prostate cancer screening?

Prostate cancer screening is of maximal benefit for men who are going to live long enough to experience the benefits of treatment, typically, survival for at least ten years from the diagnosis of prostate cancer. Thus, if you have medical conditions that make survival of ten additional years less likely, you probably would not benefit from the early detection and treatment of prostate cancer and could stop prostate cancer screening. In addition, if you feel that you would not want any treatment for prostate cancer regardless of your age and overall health, then you should stop prostate cancer screening.

The American Urologic Association (AUA) advises that PSA testing should be offered to well-informed men age 40 years or older who have a life expectancy of at least 10 years.

30. What is a digital rectal examination (DRE), and who should perform the DRE?

Because the prostate gland lies in front of the rectum, the back wall of the prostate gland can be felt by putting a gloved, lubricated finger into the rectum and feeling the prostate by pressing on the anterior wall of the rectum (**Figure 6**). The rectal examination allows one to feel only the back of the prostate. Ideally, the same doctor should perform the rectal examination each year so that the doctor is able to detect subtle changes in your prostate. The exam can be performed by a urologist or by an experienced primary care provider. If the primary care provider is concerned about your examination, you will be referred to a urologist.

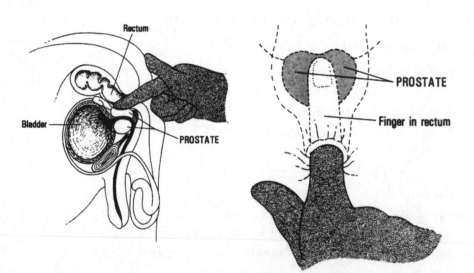

Figure 6 Digital rectal examination of the prostate.

Rous, Stephen. *The Prostate Book Sound Advice on Symptoms and Treatment*, Copyright © 1994, W.W. Norton & Co.

31. I've had my rectum removed. How can my prostate be checked?

Traditionally, prostate cancer screening involves a digital rectal examination and a serum PSA. The back surface of the prostate lies in front of the anterior surface (toward your abdomen) of the rectum; thus, pressing on the front surface of the rectum allows part of the prostate to be examined. There is no other way to physically examine the prostate. In men who have had their rectum removed for colorectal problems, such as cancer and certain inflammatory conditions, a rectal examination cannot be performed. In this situation, the physician must rely on the PSA level. If the PSA were to rise significantly, then a prostate biopsy should be performed. A transrectal ultrasound biopsy likewise cannot be performed in individuals without a rectum. In this situation, the biopsy is performed **transperineally**, which means through the **perineum** (the area under your scrotum). The ultrasound probe is placed in the area under the scrotum and in front of the expected location of the anus. The prostate is identified with the ultrasound probe, and then the needles are passed through the skin under ultrasound guidance into the different areas of the prostate. Performing biopsies this way can be more uncomfortable, and they are often performed with some form of anesthesia (general, spinal, or intravenous sedation).

Transperineal

Through the perineum.

Perineum

The area of the body that is behind the scrotum and in front of the anus.

32. What is a prostate nodule?

A prostate nodule is a firm, hard area in the prostate that feels like the knuckle of your finger. A prostate nodule may be cancerous and should be biopsied. Not all prostate nodules are cancers. Other causes of a nodule or a firm area in the prostate include prostatitis (prostate infection or inflammation), prostate calculi, an old **infarct** (an area of dead tissue resulting from a sudden loss of its blood supply) in the prostate, or abnormalities of the rectum, such as a hemorrhoid.

Infarct

An area of dead tissue resulting from a sudden loss of its blood supply.

33. If the PSA is increased, is the DRE always abnormal? And if the DRE is abnormal, is the PSA always abnormal?

When the PSA is increased, the rectal examination is not always abnormal. Remember that there are other causes of an increased PSA besides cancer. In addition, the rectal examination allows the doctor to examine only the back wall of the prostate, so some prostate cancers are not palpable by rectal examination. On the other hand, the PSA is not always increased when the rectal examination is abnormal. The PSA varies with the amount of prostate cancer present and with the grade of the cancer. In addition, a prostate nodule found during an examination is not always a cancer; it may be something in the wall of the rectum or may be related to prior inflammation or stones in the prostate. Further evaluation to rule out prostate cancer is indicated if either assessment (PSA or digital rectal examination) or both are abnormal.

34. If my PSA increases, do I need a biopsy done right away?

Because the PSA test is very sensitive and may be affected by inflammation or irritation of the prostate, the PSA value may fluctuate in some men who do not have cancer. If the rectal examination is normal, you can talk with your physician about repeating the PSA in six weeks to see whether it is returning to your baseline, or if this is your first PSA, to see whether it returns to a normal range. If it remains elevated or continues to increase, then a biopsy should be performed. Cancer cells do not sleep, they continue to grow, so there is no benefit to delaying the biopsy or subsequent treatment if the biopsy is positive. If the repeat PSA is decreasing, the PSA test could be repeated in 4 to 6 weeks, and monitoring could continue until the PSA normalizes or returns to your baseline.

35. What does a TRUS-guided prostate biopsy involve?

The transrectal ultrasound may be performed in your urologist's office or in the radiology department, depending on your institution. In preparation for the study, you may be asked to take an enema to clean stool out of the rectum and to take some antibiotics around the time of the study. You will be asked to stop taking any aspirin or nonsteroidal anti-inflammatory medications, for about one week prior to the biopsy to minimize bleeding. The doctor will ask you to lie on your side with your legs bent and brought up to your abdomen. The ultrasound probe, which is a little larger than your thumb, is then gently placed into the rectum. This can cause some transient discomfort that usually stops when the probe is in place and completely goes away when the probe is removed. Men who have had prior rectal surgery, who have active hemorrhoids, or who are very anxious and cannot relax the external sphincter muscle may have more discomfort. Once the probe is in a good position, the prostate will be evaluated to make sure that there are no suspicious areas on the ultrasound.

Ultrasound looks at tissues by sound waves. The probe emits the sound waves, and the waves hit the prostate and are bounced off the prostate and surrounding tissue. The waves then return to the ultrasound probe, and a picture is developed on the screen. The sound waves do not cause any discomfort. Prostate cancer tends to cause less reflection of the sound waves, a trait referred to as **hypoechoic**, so the area often looks different in an ultrasound image than the normal prostate tissue. After the prostate has been evaluated, biopsies are obtained. The transrectal ultrasound allows the urologist to visualize the location for the biopsies. A minimum of six to eight biopsies are obtained and more frequently twelve distributed between the top, the bottom, and the middle aspect of the prostate on each side. If you have a large prostate gland, have suspicious areas on ultrasound, or have had prior negative prostate biopsies, more biopsies may be obtained.

36. Who decides that prostate cancer is present?

After your prostate biopsies have been obtained, they are sent to the **pathologist**, a doctor who specializes in the diagnosis of disease by studying cells and tissues under the microscope. The pathologist looks at the cells in the prostate biopsy specimens under the microscope to see if they appear normal or not. The pathologist may identify normal-appearing prostate cells, prostatitis (inflammation or infection of the prostate), benign prostatic enlargement, or cancerous cells. If cancerous cells are present, then the pathologist will look closely at the cells and assign a Gleason grade and score. The Gleason grading system helps describe the appearance of the cancerous cells and may affect your **prognosis**

Hypoechoic

In ultrasonography, giving off few echoes; said of tissues or structures that reflect relatively few ultrasound waves directed at them.

Pathologist

A doctor trained in the evaluation of tissues under the microscope to determine the presence/absence of disease.

Prognosis

The long-term outlook or prospect for survival and recovery from a disease.

The Gleason grading system helps describe the appearance of the cancerous cells and may affect your prognosis (the prediction made as to the outcome of your disease). In addition to the Gleason grade and score, the pathologist will also comment on how much of each biopsy specimen had prostate cancer cells in it; this, too, may affect your prognosis (see Question 38).

37. Can the pathologist make a mistake in the diagnosis?

The use of a common grading system helps maintain uniformity in the grading of prostate cancer. The interobserver agreement (agreement between two different pathologists) and the intraobserver agreement (the same pathologist arriving at the same conclusion after reviewing the same slide twice) for the Gleason grading system are more than 80% and 90%, respectively. This means that two different pathologists reviewing the same slide agree on the Gleason grade for that slide 80% of the time, and that the same pathologist reviewing the same slide twice assigns the same grade to it both times 90% of the time.

The most frequent cause of differences in grading is the grading of tumors that vary between two grades. A Gleason sum of 2 to 4 is uncommon and should be found only in a small number of needle biopsy specimens. It is the Gleason sum of 2 to 4 that tends to be upgraded to a higher sum a small percentage of the time when reviewed by another pathologist. There is a tendency for the needle biopsy Gleason grade to be lower than the pathologic grade at the time of radical prostatectomy. This difference in Gleason grade probably reflects the presence of a higher-grade cancer in another area of the prostate that had not been biopsied at the time of the prostate biopsy. It is very rare for the pathologist to say that there is no cancer in the specimen and for another pathologist to state that there is. (Similarly, it is rare for one pathologist to say that cancer is present and another pathologist to state that it is not present).

38. What is the Gleason grade/score?

The grade of a cancer is a term used to describe how the cancer cells look; that is, whether the cells look aggressive and not very similar to normal cells (high grade) or whether they look very similar to normal cells (low grade). The grade of the cancer is an important factor in predicting long-term results of treatment, response to treatment, and survival. With prostate cancer, the most commonly used grading system is the **Gleason scale**. In this grading system, cells are examined by a pathologist under the microscope and assigned a number based on how the cancer cells look and how they are arranged together (**Figure 7**). Because prostate cancer may be composed of cancer cells of different grades, the pathologist assigns numbers to the two predominant grades present. The numbers range from 1 (low grade) to 5 (high grade). Typically, the Gleason score is the total of these two numbers; for example, a man with a Gleason grade of 2 and 3 in his prostate cancer would have a Gleason score of 5. An exception to this occurs where the highest (most aggressive) pattern present in a biopsy is neither the most predominant nor the second most predominant pattern. In this situation, the Gleason score is obtained by combining the most predominant pattern grade with the highest grade. Occasionally, if a small component of a tumor on prostatectomy is of a pattern that is higher than the two most predominant patterns, then the minor component is noted as a tertiary grade to the pathology report.

Gleason scale

A commonly used method to classify how cells appear in cancerous tissues; the less the cancerous cells look like normal cells, the more malignant the cancer; two numbers, each from 1 to 5, are assigned to the two most predominant types of cells present. These two numbers are added together to produce the Gleason score. Higher numbers indicate more aggressive cancers.

PROSTATIC ADENOCARCINOMA
(Histologic Grades)

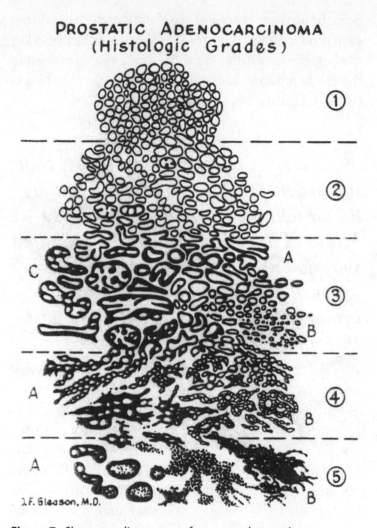

Figure 7 Gleason grading system of prostate adenocarcinoma.
Reprinted with permission from JI Epstein, *Campbell's Urology*, (7th Ed), Copyright © 1997 W. B. Saunders Co.

Low-score cancers are those with a Gleason score of 2, 3, or 4. Intermediate-score cancers are those with a Gleason score of 5, 6, or 7. And high-score cancers are those with a Gleason score of 8, 9, or 10. The speed of growth and the aggressiveness of the cancer increase with the Gleason score. Gleason scores 8 through 10 are highly aggressive tumors that are often difficult to cure.

Sometimes these cancers are so abnormal that they do not even produce PSA. The grade of the cancer identified by the biopsies may differ from the grade that is present in the entire prostate, because it is possible that the biopsy may not identify areas of higher-grade cancers.

39. I recently had a prostate biopsy that showed no prostate cancer cells, but my doctor tells me I need a repeat biopsy because I have PIN. What is PIN and why do I need a repeat biopsy?What are atypical glands suspicious for prostate cancer? Do I need a repeat biopsy with this finding?

PIN (prostatic intraepithelial neo-plasia)

An abnormal area in a prostate biopsy specimen that is not cancerous, but may become cancerous or be associated with cancer else where in the prostate.

PIN is the abbreviation for **prostatic intraepithelial neoplasia**. PIN is identified by the pathologist examining the prostate biopsies. PIN has been thought to be a precancerous lesion. More recently, PIN has been divided into two types, low-grade PIN and high-grade PIN, based on how the cells look. Low-grade PIN does not appear to have any increased risk of prostate cancer. High-grade PIN, however, is often found in association with prostate cancer. In 35–45% of men who undergo a repeat biopsy for high-grade PIN, prostate cancer cells are present in the repeat biopsy. If your doctor has performed multiple biopsies (i.e., 10–12) then the recommendation is to consider a delayed repeat biopsy. If your doctor only did six biopsies, then an immediate repeat biopsy is indicated. Atypical gland; suspicious for cancer is noted on the pathology report when the pathologist sees an atypical area that has most of the features of cancer, but a definitive diagnosis of cancer cannot be made due to the small size of the area and the small number of abnormal cells present. Repeat biopsy in patients with this diagnosis have up to a 60% chance of having prostate cancer present in a repeat biopsy. Thus, the finding of atypical gland; suspicious for cancer warrants an immediate rebiopsy (within 3 months) with increased number of biopsies from the abnormal area and the areas nearby. If no cancer is found on the repeat biopsy then close follow-up with PSA, digital rectal examination and periodic biopsy may be needed. See http://www.pccnc.org/early_detection/2004_NCCD_guidelines.pdf

40. I just had a TURP, and my doctor called and told me that there is cancer in the specimen. Will the TURP cause my cancer to spread? Will it prevent me from having certain treatments for prostate cancer?

Before the identification of PSA, prostate cancer was detected by a palpable nodule on digital rectal examination, the presence of metastatic disease, or transurethral resection of the prostate, also called transurethral prostatectomy (TURP). TURP is one of the most common forms of surgical therapy for benign hyperplasia of the prostate (BPH). The procedure uses an instrument called a resectoscope (similar to a telescope—it has an eyepiece, a lens, and a light source), which is passed through the urethra. The prostatic tissue that is bulging into the urethra and blocking the outflow of urine is cut away (resected) using a special loop that is connected to an electrical current. The resection is continued until it appears that all of the obstructing prostate tissue is removed. The prostate tissue, called "chips," is then removed through the scope and sent to the pathologist for examination under a microscope.

Similar to the procedure with needle biopsies of the prostate, if the pathologist identifies cancer cells in the specimen, he or she grades the prostate cancer cells and determines a Gleason score. The pathologist also determines what percentage of the prostate chips have cancer present in them. Typically, if less than 5% of the chips contain cancer and the Gleason score is low (< 6), then the prostate cancer is considered to be clinically insignificant, and you can be followed with digital rectal examinations and PSA tests. If more than 5% of the tissue contains prostate cancer and/or the Gleason score is high, the cancer is considered to be potentially aggressive and warrants further treatment. Similar to any newly diagnosed prostate cancer, it is important to determine the clinical stage of the cancer and to assess whether the cancer is likely to be confined to the prostate through the use of tables, such as the **Partin Table** (**Tables 5** and **6**), and staging studies, such as a bone scan, if indicated.

The TURP does not cause the prostate cancer to spread, nor does it make it easier for the cancer cells to spread. However, the TURP can affect the risks of future treatments for prostate cancer. A TURP makes interstitial seed therapy more difficult to perform and is associated with a much higher risk of urinary incontinence, making it less desirable. Radical prostatectomy and external-beam radiation therapy can be performed after TURP without an increased risk.

Partin tables

Tables that are developed based on results of the PSA, clinical stage, and Gleason score involving thousands of men with prostate cancer. These tables are used to predict the likelihood that prostate cancer has spread to the lymph nodes or seminal vesicles, penetrated the capsule, or remains confined to the prostate. The tables were developed by Dr. Partin at Johns Hopkins University.

Table 5 Multivariate Logistic Regression Analysis for Prediction of Pathologic Stage Using Prostate-Specific Antigen, Gleason Score, and Clinical Stage (TNM): Prediction of Organ-Confined Disease (Percent)

Prostate-Specific Antigen Level (ng/mL)

	0.0–4.0 Clinical Stage							4.1–10.0 Clinical Stage						
Score	T1a	T1b	T1c	T2a	T2b	T2c	T3a	T1a	T1b	T1c	T2a	T2b	T2c	T3a
2–4	100	85	92	88	76	82	—	100	78	82	83	67	71	—
5	100	78	81	81	67	73	—	100	70	71	73	56	64	43
6	100	68	69	72	54	60	42	100	53	59	62	44	48	33
7	—	54	55	61	41	46	—	100	39	43	51	32	37	26
8–10	—	—	—	48	31	—	—	—	32	31	39	22	25	12

Prostate-Specific Antigen Level (ng/mL)

	10.0–20.0 Clinical Stage							>20 Clinical Stage						
Score	T1a	T1b	T1c	T2a	T2b	T2c	T3a	T1a	T1b	T1c	T2a	T2b	T2c	T3a
2–4	100	—	—	61	52	—	—	—	—	33	20	7	—	—
5	100	49	55	58	43	37	26	—	—	24	32	—	3	—
6	—	36	41	44	28	37	19	—	—	22	14	1	4	5
7	—	24	24	36	19	24	14	—	—	7	18	4	5	3
8–10	—	11	—	29	14	15	9	—	—	3	3	—	2	2

Table 6 Multivariate Logistic Regression Analysis For Prediction of Pathologic Stage Using Prostate-Specific Antigen, Gleason Score, and Clinical Stage (TNM); Prediction of Lymph Nodal Status (Percent)

Prostate-Specific Antigen Level (ng/mL)

0.0–4.0 Clinical Stage

Score	T1a	T1b	T1c	T2a	T2b	T2c	T3a
2–4	0	2	<1	1	2	4	—
5	0	4	1	2	4	8	—
6	0	8	2	3	9	17	15
7	—	15	2	7	18	31	—
8–10	—	—	—	13	32	—	—

4.1–10.0 Clinical Stage

Score	T1a	T1b	T1c	T2a	T2b	T2c	T3a
2–4	0	2	1	1	2	5	—
5	0	4	1	2	5	10	8
6	0	9	2	4	11	19	16
7	0	18	3	8	20	34	28
8–10	—	30	5	15	35	53	50

Prostate-Specific Antigen Level (ng/mL)

10.0–20.0 Clinical Stage

Score	T1a	T1b	T1c	T2a	T2b	T2c	T3a
2–4	0	—	—	1	3	—	—
5	0	5	3	2	6	13	11
6	—	11	4	5	13	22	20
7	—	21	7	9	24	39	35
8–10	—	41	—	17	40	59	54

> 20 Clinical Stage

Score	T1a	T1b	T1c	T2a	T2b	T2c	T3a
2–4	—	—	6	2	7	—	—
5	—	—	9	3	—	29	—
6	—	—	8	9	18	53	31
7	—	—	24	11	44	62	55
8–10	—	—	41	35	76	73	65

Reprinted with permission from H. B. Carter and A. W. Partin, *Campbell's Urology* (7th Ed.), Copyright © 1997 W. B. Saunders Co.

PART FOUR

Prostate Cancer Staging

How does one know if the prostate cancer
is confined to the prostate?

How and why does one stage prostate cancer?

What is a bone scan?

More . . .

41. How does one know if the prostate cancer is confined to the prostate?

By staging your cancer, your doctor is trying to assess, based on your prostate biopsy results, your physical examination, your PSA, and other tests and X-rays (if obtained), whether your prostate cancer is confined to the prostate, and if it is not, to what extent it has spread. Studies of large numbers of men who have undergone radical prostatectomy and pelvic lymph node dissections have established some guidelines regarding the likelihood of prostate capsular involvement and lymph node metastases (Tables 5 and 6). It was initially thought that magnetic resonance imaging (MRI) would be very helpful in determining whether capsular penetration and extracapsular disease were present; however, it has only proved to be useful in centers that perform large numbers of MRIs. Similarly, the use of computed tomographic (CT) scanning in assessing whether or not the cancer has spread to the pelvic lymph nodes has been disappointing (see Question 42).

42. How and why does one stage prostate cancer?

Knowing the stage (the size and the extent of spread) of the prostate cancer helps the doctor counsel you on treatment options. Your doctor may tell you a "clinical" stage (**Figure 8**), based on your rectal examination, prostate biopsies, and radiographic/nuclear medicine studies (CT scan, bone scan, MRI). Pathological staging is performed when a pathologist examines the prostate, seminal vesicles, and pelvic lymph nodes (if removed) at the time of radical prostatectomy. The most common staging system used is called the **TNM System**. In this

TNM System

The most common staging system for prostate cancer. It reflects the size of the tumor, nodal disease, and metastatic disease.

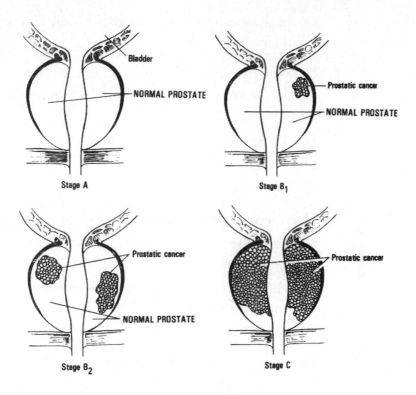

Figure 8 The prostate gland showing the different stages of cancer.
Rous, Stephen. *The Prostate Book Sound Advice on Symptoms and Treatment,* Copyright © 1994, W. W. Norton & Co., p. 91.

system, T refers to the size of the **tumor** in the prostate, N refers to the extent of cancerous involvement of the lymph nodes, and M refers to the presence or absence of **metastases** (deposits of prostate cancer outside of the prostate and lymph nodes).

T   Refers to the size of the tumor in the prostate

T1   The prostate cancer is located within the prostate and cannot be palpated on rectal examination

T1a: tumor is found incidentally in < 5% of the prostate tissue, such as during a TURP

T1b: tumor is found incidentally in > 5% of the prostate tissue, such as during a TURP

Tumor

Abnormal tissue growth that may be cancerous or noncancerous (benign).

Metastases

See Metastatic Cancer.

47

T1c: prostate cancer is identified by needle biopsy for an increased PSA

T2 The prostate cancer is still located in the prostate and the tumor is large enough to be felt on rectal examination

T2a: tumor involves half of a lobe or less

T2b: tumor involves one lobe

T2c: tumor involves both lobes

T3 The tumor extends through the prostate capsule

T3a: tumor has spread outside of the prostate capsule on one side

T3b: tumor has spread outside of the prostate capsule on both sides

T3c: tumor invades one or both seminal vesicles

T4 The tumor is fixed or invades adjacent structures other than seminal vesicles, such as bladder neck, external sphincter, rectum, levator muscles, and/or pelvic wall

T4a: tumor invades bladder neck and/or external sphincter and/or rectum

T4b: tumor invades levator muscles and/or is fixed to pelvic side wall

N Describes the extent of lymph node involvement

N0: no evidence of any metastases in the pelvic lymph nodes

N1: prostate cancer cells found in a single, small (<2 cm) lymph node

N2: prostate cancer found in a single larger (>2 cm but <5 cm) lymph node or in several lymph nodes <5 cm in size

N3: lymph node metastases that are >5 cm in size

M   Refers to the presence or absence of metastases

>   *M0:* no evidence of distant metastases (tumor outside of the pelvis)

>   *M1:* distant metastases (tumor spread outside of the pelvis to other areas of the body, such as bones, liver)

The other staging system that is often used is the **Whitmore-Jewett System**.

Stage A: no clinical evidence of tumor

>   *A1:* tumor found incidentally at TURP with < 5% of the tissue removed at TURP having cancer in it

>   *A2:* tumor found incidentally at TURP with > 5% of the tissue removed having cancer in it

Stage B: palpable tumor that is confined within the prostate gland

>   *B1N:* tumor involve ≤ ½ lobe and is surrounded by normal tissue

>   *B1:* tumor involves < 1 lobe

>   *B2:* tumor involves ≥ 1 lobe

Stage C: tumor extends through the prostate capsule

>   *C1:* palpable tumor extending through the prostate capsule (unilateral or bilateral) and/or involving seminal vesicle(s), tumor , 6 cm in diameter

>   *C2:* tumor ≥ 6 cm in diameter, may be fixed or invade adjacent structures other than seminal vesicles

Stage D: metastatic disease

>   *D0:* elevation of prostatic acid phosphatase only

>   *D1:* pelvic lymph node metastases

Whitmore-Jewett System

An alternative staging system for prostate cancer.

D1.5: increasing PSA after failed local therapy

D2: distant metastases

D2.5: increasing PSA after nadir level D3: hormone-refractory prostate cancer

D3.5: hormonally sensitive prostate cancer (resistant to orchiectomy or LHRH analogues, but sensitive to other hormonal manipulations)

D4: hormonally insensitive (resistant to all hormonal manipulation)

43. What is a bone scan?

Bone scan

A specialized nuclear medicine study that allows one to detect changes in the bone that may be related to metastatic prostate cancer.

A **bone scan** is a study performed in the nuclear medicine department that involves injecting a small amount of a radioactive chemical through a vein into your bloodstream. The chemical circulates through your body and is picked up by areas of fast bone growth that may be associated with cancer. The bone scan is the most sensitive technique currently available for identifying prostate cancer that has spread to the bones. Other problems of the bones, such as a history of a broken bone, arthritis, and a condition called Paget's disease, may cause an increase in uptake of the radioactive chemical. Often, your history, the location of the bone, and possible additional studies, such as a plain X-ray study or an MRI, will help determine whether the area of increased uptake indicates the presence of cancer.

The bone scan is quite sensitive, but it does not identify small numbers of cancer cells in the bones. In a small number of men (8%), the bone scan may be normal when bone metastases are present. Prostate cancer is not the only cancer that spreads to the bone, but prostate cancer tends to cause the bone to look different than that of involvement with other cancers, such as breast, colon, and bladder. Prostate cancer metastases are typically osteoblastic, whereas those of other cancers tend to be osteolytic. **Osteoblastic lesions** look as if there is an increase in the amount of bone present on a plain X-ray, whereas **osteolytic lesions** look like there is a loss of bone. The bone scan may also show obstruction of the urinary tract, leading to hydronephrosis (a back-up of urine in the kidney that causes swelling of the kidney).

The bone scan is often obtained as part of the staging work-up in men with prostate cancer and is helpful in men with a rising PSA (either after primary treatment, such as radical prostatectomy, or during watchful waiting) with or without bone pain to identify new areas of uptake that may indicate new bone involvement. The bone scan is usually obtained as part of the staging evaluation in men with newly diagnosed prostate cancer who have a PSA > 10 ng/mL. Because the risk of bone metastases in men with newly diagnosed prostate cancer who have a PSA < 10 ng/mL is so low, a bone scan is not routinely obtained in these men. Although the chemical used for the study is radioactive, the amount used is small, and it will not put you or your family at risk.

Osteoblastic lesion

Pertaining to plain X-ray of a bone, increased density of bone seen on X-ray when there is extensive new bone formation due to cancerous destruction of the bone.

Osteolytic lesion

Pertaining to plain X-ray of a bone, refers to decreased density of bone seen on X-ray when there is destruction and loss of bone by cancer.

44. What is a pelvic lymph node dissection and what are the risks?

The first location to which prostate cancer tends to spread if it goes outside of the prostate is the pelvic lymph nodes. It is important to know whether the cancer has spread to the lymph nodes because the success rates of treatments such as interstitial seed therapy and radical prostatectomy are lower if the cancer has spread into the pelvic lymph nodes. Thus, the urologist or radiation oncologist should have a good idea whether there is prostate cancer involvement of the pelvic lymph nodes before recommending a therapy. Unfortunately, radio-logic studies such as CT scans have not been helpful in identifying individuals with smaller amounts of cancer in the pelvic lymph nodes. The most accurate way to assess the lymph node status is to remove the lymph nodes and have them examined by the pathologist. The lymph nodes to which prostate cancer typically spreads are located in the lateral aspect of each side of the pelvis (see Question 22). Removing the lymph nodes requires surgery, either an open procedure or a laparoscopic procedure, which has risks. The use of the ProstaScint scan (see Question 45) to detect prostate cancer in the pelvic lymph nodes is being evaluated.

Not everyone needs a pelvic lymph node dissection. When the risk of having positive lymph nodes is low, such as occurs in men with a low Gleason score or a PSA < 10, a lymph node dissection is unnecessary, and one can proceed directly with definitive therapy, such as interstitial seed therapy, external beam radiation therapy (EBRT), and radical prostatectomy (see Part 5, *Treatment of Prostate Cancer*, for descriptions of these therapies). In high-risk patients, those with higher Gleason scores (8–10), or those with a PSA > 10, a lymph node dissection may be performed at the same time as a planned radical prostatectomy or before planned EBRT or interstitial seed therapy. If an open prostatectomy or laparoscopic robotic prostatectomy is planned, the lymph nodes can be removed using the same approach as for the prostatectomy and can be examined by the pathologist (frozen section) just before the prostatectomy. Frozen section specimens are interpreted by the pathologist shortly after they are removed from the patient, and the findings are reported to the surgeon in the operating room.

The surgeon then decides whether to proceed with removal of the prostate based on whether cancer has been identified in the lymph nodes. Some surgeons remove the prostate in the presence of small amounts of cancer in the lymph nodes, whereas others do not. The slides are then made into permanent sections and reviewed again by the pathologist. In most cases, the interpretation of the frozen section is the same as that of the permanent section; rarely do the two differ. In a perineal prostatectomy, the perineal incision does not allow access to the pelvic lymph nodes, and a separate midline incision or a laparoscopic approach is needed for the lymph node dissection. With EBRT or interstitial seed therapy, the pelvic lymph node dissection may be performed laparoscopically or via an open incision that is located below the umbilicus on a separate day before EBRT/interstitial seeds.

A lymph node dissection should be performed in high-risk patients because it may affect treatment. The likelihood of having positive nodes varies with the stage of the prostate cancer, the PSA value, and the Gleason score. Approximately 5–12% of men who are believed to have clinically localized prostate cancer (low stage) have cancer that has spread to the pelvic lymph nodes. Before the pelvic lymph node dissection, you should discuss with your doctor how your planned prostate cancer treatment would be affected if you had cancer involving the pelvic lymph nodes.

The main risks of a pelvic lymph node dissection are bleeding, nerve injury, and lymphocele.

- *Bleeding:* The nodes that are removed at the time of the pelvic lymph node dissection surround some large pelvic arteries and veins, called the iliac vessels. Injury to these vessels or their branches may cause bleeding. It is rare to have a significant blood loss such that a blood transfusion would be required.

- *Nerve injury:* The obturator nerve supplies muscles in the leg and is surrounded by some of the pelvic lymph nodes. If the nerve is cut or damaged at the time of surgery and the damage is recognized, it may be sewn back together. If the injury is not recognized, it may lead to permanent inability to cross your leg on the side of the injury.

- *Lymphocele:* A lymphocele is a collection of lymph fluid that accumulates in the pelvis. Lymphoceles result from injury to the lymph vessels. When the lymph nodes are being removed, the lymphatic vessels are clipped, tied, or cauterized to minimize leakage of lymph fluid from the vessel. A lymphocele may go undetected and may not cause any harm. If the lymphocele gets large enough, it may put pressure on other tissues and cause abdominal pressure or pain. If the lymphocele becomes infected, you may develop a fever or chills and abdominal pain. Lymphoceles are identified in one to two of every 100 men undergoing radical prostatectomy. The actual incidence may be higher with smaller lymphoceles that do not cause any symptoms and thus are not identified. Treatment of a lymphocele varies with its size and symptoms. If the lymphocele is small and does not cause any symptoms, it can be monitored to see whether it will go away on its own. If the lymphocele is large and causes symptoms or if it is infected, then it should be drained. Usually, a radiologist is able to pass a small drainage tube through the skin into the area where the lymphocele is located to drain the fluid. The drain is left in place until there is no further drainage and an ultrasound or CT scan shows that the lymphocele has resolved. In most patients, this is all that is needed. Rarely, the lymphocele recurs, requiring repeat drainage or surgery.

45. What is a ProstaScint scan?

The ProstaScint scan is a relatively new nuclear medicine scan that is similar to a bone scan. Unlike the bone scan, it looks primarily at the tissues to see whether prostate cancer has spread in these areas. It may be helpful to identify areas of recurrent prostate cancer after surgery if the PSA is increasing and the bone scan is negative. Some studies suggest that the ProstaScint scan may also be helpful in the initial staging of prostate cancer. These studies have demonstrated that the ProstaScint scan is more sensitive and specific than a CT scan and MRI in the detection of pelvic lymph node involvement with prostate cancer. However, it is not currently being used as part of the initial staging work-up in all cases. Interpretation of the ProstaScint scan requires a skilled nuclear medicine radiologist.

PART FIVE

Treatment of Prostate Cancer

Why do I need a team of doctors to treat me?
Who are they?

What options do I have for treatment
of my prostate cancer?

How do I decide which treatment is best for me?

More . . .

46. Why do I need a team of doctors to treat me? Who are they?

Cancer is a complex disease, and understanding and treating it requires knowledge of genetics, molecular biology, pharmacology, radiation therapy, nutrition, surgery, and other essential information. No one doctor is able to provide all the care and service you may need, so it's necessary that a team of specialists look at your case from the perspective of each clinician's area of expertise.

You may wish to talk with your urologist about making a *medical oncologist* part of your treatment team. This multidisciplinary approach will ensure that you have access to all of the treatment options available. The following doctors are likely to play a role on your team:

Urologist: A urologist specializes in the diagnosis and treatment of disorders of the genito-urinary system. Your urologist probably diagnosed your prostate cancer and helped you plan your course of treatment. This physician has likely been overseeing all your procedures and program of therapy.

Radiation oncologist: This type of doctor treats cancer through radiation, or high-energy rays. You might have received radiation therapy from a radiation oncologist in the form of external beam radiation or brachytherapy. External beam radiation directs X-rays from a machine at the prostate gland. Brachytherapy consists of tiny radioactive seeds placed inside or near the tumor (see Question 47).

Medical oncologist: If prostate cancer reappears despite surgery or no longer responds to hormonal therapy, a medical oncologist should join the treatment team because he or she may use chemotherapy. A medical oncologist is a doctor who specializes in treating patients diagnosed with cancer. He or she helps you plan chemotherapy and takes

Urologist

A doctor that specializes in the evaluation and treatment of diseases of the genito-urinary tract in men and women.

Radiation oncologist

A physician who treats cancer through the use of radiation therapy.

Medical oncologist

See oncologist.

charge of chemotherapy treatment. The medical oncologist may also make recommendations regarding clinical trials (see Question 89).

47. What options do I have for treatment of my prostate cancer?

Cliff's comment:

After finally realizing that despite feeling great, I did indeed have prostate cancer, I had to figure out what the best treatment for me was. When faced with the option of leaving my prostate in place or removing it, I knew that, even though I was petrified of surgery, it would be the best thing for me in the long run. I knew that I could not live with my prostate gland and the continuous question of whether there were any viable cancer cells remaining in my prostate after interstitial seeds or radiation therapy.

Palliative

Treatment designed to relieve a particular problem without necessarily solving it, e.g., palliative therapy is given in order to relieve symptoms and improve quality of life, but it does not cure the patient.

Various treatment options are available for prostate cancer, each with its own risks and benefits (**Table 7**). The options available may vary with the grade of tumor, the extent of tumor spread, your overall medical health and life expectancy and your personal preferences. The treatments for prostate cancer can be divided into those that are intended to "cure" your cancer (definitive therapies) and those that are **palliative**, intended to slow down the growth of the prostate cancer and treat its symptoms. Definitive therapies for localized prostate cancer include: interstitial seed therapy (brachytherapy), external beam radiation (EBRT) and radical prostatectomy (either open, laparoscopic or robotic). Other therapies, such as cryotherapy, high intensity focused ultrasound (HIFU) and combination therapy (external beam radiation plus interstitial seed therapy) are not commonly used for men with localized prostate cancer.

The treatments for prostate cancer can be divided into those that are intended to "cure" your cancer (definitive therapies) and those that are palliative, intended to slow down the growth of the prostate cancer and treat its symptoms.

Table 7 Treatment Options for Prostate Cancer

Mode of Treatment	Advantages	Disadvantages	Curative: Yes/No	Alternative If Fails
Hormonal therapy • Therapy in which the male hormones (androgens) are eliminated from the body. • Primary treatment for older men with prostate cancer who don't want surgery or forms of XRT but also don't want to watch and wait. • Also used as therapy for men with metastatic disease.	1. Orchiectomy: A one time procedure that avoids the need for shots; it drops testosterone quickly to almost zero and is permanent. 2. LHRH analogues: Not permanent. 3. LHRH antagonist: Not permanent; no flare phenomenon. 4. Antiandrogen therapy: Diarrhea, liver damage, impaired night vision.	1. Orchiectomy: Permanent outpatient procedure involves minor surgery, risk of infection, bleeding, pain. 2. LHRH analogue: Can have flair of bone pain in those with bone metastases; need to pretreat these men with androgen receptor blocker; requires every one month to yearly visits/or shots, which can be expensive. 3. LHRH antagonist: Requires monthly shots throughout the year; can be expensive. 4. Antiandrogen therapy: Blocks cells' ability to absorb the hormone often used in conjunction with shots. Most antiandrogens are not effective as a single agent, however.	No: hormone therapy stops the growth of those prostate cancer cells that are hormone sensitive. Used for treatment of metastatic diagnosis.	Chemotherapy

Mode of Treatment	Advantages	Disadvantages	Curative: Yes/No	Alternative If Fails
Cryotherapy/ Surgery	Minimally invasive, no blood loss. Quicker recovery; one-time procedure; can be used in those who cannot undergo RRPX or as salvage procedure for local recurrence after XRT.	Impotence, urethral strictures, urinary retention, urinary frequency, dysuria, hematuria, penile or scrotal swelling, fistula, incomplete treatment of cancer. Works better on smaller prostates; more difficult to perform if prior TURP (transurethral resection of prostate); incontinence up to 30% when used as salvage procedure.	Role is not well defined; this therapy is being used primarily for XRT failures, but some have used it as 1st line.	Hormone treatment, radical prostatectomy, but there is increased risk of complicatio
Radical retropubic prostatectomy with/without bilateral pelvic lymph node dissection (open)	One-time procedure that may cure prostate cancer in earlier stages. Allows for pathologic staging of disease. PSA goes to undetectable if no remaining prostate cancer.	Incontinence; impotence; bladder neck contracture. Rarely: a need for blood transfusion, nerve injury, rectal injury. Longer recovery period, 2–4% incidence of permanent incontinence. 20–40% incidence of permanent impotence.	Yes, in setting of localized diagnosis.	If it fails locally, external beam radiation therapy is used. If it fails in distant disease (metastases), hormones are used.

(continues)

Table 7 Treatment Options for Prostate Cancer (Continued)

Mode of Treatment	Advantages	Disadvantages	Curative: Yes/No	Alternative If Fails
External beam radiation therapy	Avoids major surgery; may cure prostate cancer in early stages. Incontinence and impotence less common than with surgery. No transfusion risk.	Fatigue; skin reaction in treated areas; urinary frequency and dysuria; proctitis, rectal bleeding, frequent stools, urgency; bowel function may remain abnormal; hematuria. Rare: fistula. No lymph node analysis or pathologic staging; requires treatments 5 days a week for 6 to 7 weeks; 30–50% chance of erectile dysfunction; 10–15% chance of bladder and/or rectal irritation. May have hair loss in area receiving full dose such as pubic hair. PSA doesn't go to undetectable levels.	Yes, in setting of localized diagnosis.	Hormone treatment, which is palliative. Salvage prostatectomy with associated increased risk of incontinence.
Laparoscopic radical prostatectomy & robotic-assisted radical prostatectomy	Quicker recovery; less postoperative pain; possible better visualization of pelvic anatomy. Allows for accurate staging; same advantages as RRPX. Less blood loss compared to open radical prostatectomy. Robotic vs. lap—faster OR time, easier to perform. Comparable short-term outcomes to open surgery	Laparoscopic A long procedure that was first pioneered by French in 1998; long-term data not available. Steep learning curve. Robot is extremely expensive.	Yes, if localized diagnosis.	Locally, XRT; in distant disease, hormones are used.

Mode of Treatment	Advantages	Disadvantages	Curative: Yes/No	Alternative If Fails
Brachytherapy (interstitial seeds)	Minimally invasive; quick recovery, short hospitalization; no transfusions.	This therapy is not for every patient (men with high grade cancer, PSA > 10, Gleason score ≥ 7, are more likely to fail). Large glands are more difficult. Urinary frequency, urgency, hematuria, rectal irritation, pain, burning, frequency and urgency with bowel movements. Chance of impotence or pain with ejaculation; 25–60% chance of impotence; urinary retention; harder to do if have had prior TURP.	Over the short term, if the diagnosis is localized, brachytherapy appears to be curative; long-term data need to be reviewed.	Salvage prostatectomy if localized; hormones if distant disease.
Chemotherapy	1. Kills a/o reduces growth of cancer. 2. Provides palliation (symptom relief).	Potentially significant side effects.	Some chemotherapy combinations have been shown to improve outcomes and significantly prolong survival.	

Palliative therapies for prostate cancer include the use of hormonal therapies and radiation therapy for symptomatic bone metastases. In those individuals whose prostate cancer is refractory to hormonal therapy, chemotherapy may be an option.

The option of **watchful waiting** and **active surveillance** can also be chosen. Watchful waiting involves no treatment initially. Rather, your prostate cancer is monitored with periodic PSAs and DREs and possibly X-rays. The premise of watchful waiting is that some individuals will not benefit from definitive treatment for their prostate cancer. With watchful waiting, palliative treatment (treatment designed to slow down the growth of the cancer and to treat symptoms, but not cure the cancer) is instituted for local or metastatic progression, if it occurs. Palliative therapies include: trimming of the prostate (transurethral prostatectomy) if the prostate becomes large enough that it causes trouble urinating, hormonal therapy to decrease the size and growth of the prostate cancer and radiation therapy if symptomatic bone metastases occur (see Question 83).

Active surveillance differs from watchful waiting. The goal of active surveillance is to give definitive (curative) treatment to those men with prostate cancers that are likely to progress and to decrease the risk of treatment-related side effects in those men whose cancers are less likely to progress. Thus with active surveillance one also undergoes periodic PSAs and DREs, but definitive therapy is instituted when pre-defined changes are noted. There are no established active surveillance protocols, although studies are ongoing. You and your doctor would need to discuss a mutually agreeable protocol before starting active surveillance.

Watchful waiting

Active observation and regular monitoring of a patient without actual treatment.

Active surveillance

A form of prostate cancer therapy whereby no definitive treatment is instituted initially, but definitive therapy is instituted when predefined changes are noted.

Monitoring with active surveillance is often more frequent than with watchful waiting. Active surveillance is better for older patients with shorter life expectancies and with lower risk prostate cancers

Surgery is currently the most commonly performed treatment with the intent to cure prostate cancer. The surgical procedure is called a radical prostatectomy (see Question 52) and involves the removal of the entire prostate gland. Radical prostatectomy may be performed through an **incision** (the cutting of the skin at the beginning of surgery) that extends from the umbilicus to the pubic bone (**Figure 9**), through a perineal incision (between the scrotum and the anus) (**Figure 10**), laparoscopically (**Figure 11**), and more recently with the assistance of a robot. The choice of technique varies with the patient's body characteristics and the urologist's preference.

Interstitial seed placement (**brachytherapy**) is a procedure that is gaining in popularity as it is minimally invasive and requires a single treatment. Similar to radical prostatectomy, it is a procedure with intent to cure. This procedure involves the **percutaneous** (through the skin) placement of radioactive seeds into the prostate (see Question 58, **Figure 12**). Depending on the prostate cancer grade and stage and the PSA, conformal external-beam radiation therapy (EBRT), in which beams of high-energy radiation are aimed at the prostate (or other target organ), may be used in addition to the interstitial seeds.

Conformal EBRT is a newer way of delivering EBRT to the prostate. Through the use of CT scanning and the improved ability to focus the maximum radiation effects

Incision

Cutting of the skin at the beginning of surgery.

Interstitial

Within an organ, such as interstitial brachytherapy, whereby radioactive seeds are placed into the prostate.

Brachytherapy

A form of radiation therapy whereby radioactive pellets are placed into the prostate.

Percutaneous

Through the skin.

Conformal EBRT

EBRT that uses CT scan images to better visualize radiation targets and normal tissues.

Surgery is currently the most commonly performed treatment with the intent to cure prostate cancer. The surgical procedure is called a radical prostatectomy and involves the removal of the entire prostate gland.

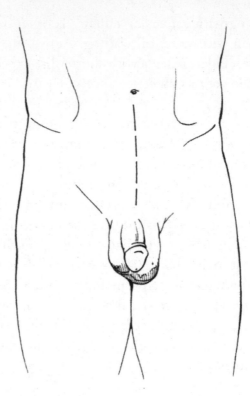

Figure 9 Surgical incision for radical retropubic prostatectomy. a midline incision is made from the symphysis pubis to the umbilicis.
Reprinted with permission from Graham Jr, SD, Glenn JF. Glenn's *Urologic Surgery* (5th Ed), Lippincott Williams & Wilkins, 1998, p. 1102.

on the prostate and less on the surrounding tissues, conformal EBRT may decrease side effects and improve results over those of traditional EBRT. This procedure is also performed with intent to cure.

Cryotherapy, cryosurgery

A prostate cancer therapy in which the prostate is frozen to destroy the cancer cells.

Cryotherapy is a minimally invasive procedure in which probes are percutaneously placed into the prostate under ultrasound guidance. Liquid nitrogen is administered through the probes to "freeze" and kill the cancer cells (see Question 71). Currently, this procedure is more commonly used as a second-line procedure when an individual has not responded to EBRT. It, too, is used with intent to cure.

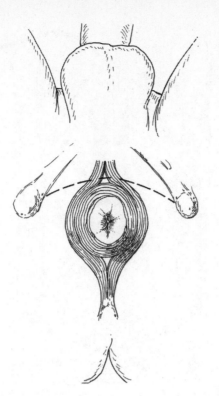

Figure 10 Radial perineal prostatectomy—incision lines.
Reprinted with permission from Gibbons RP, Radical Perineal Prostalectomy. Definitive Treatment for Patients with Localized Prostate Cancer. AUA Update Series, Volume 13, Lesson 5, AUA Office of Education, Houston, TX 1994.

High-intensity focused ultrasound (HIFU) is a procedure that is being performed in Europe and appears to be an option for lower Gleason score prostate cancers and for local recurrence of prostate cancer after external beam radiation therapy. The procedure is performed by inserting a probe into the rectum. The probe delivers highly focused ultrasound to the prostate. The high intensity focused ultrasound heats the prostate to temperatures of 80–100 degrees centigrade, which is enough to kill prostate cancer cells. The effect is limited to the prostate and does not irritate the rectal tissue. HIFU is not currently approved for use in the United States.

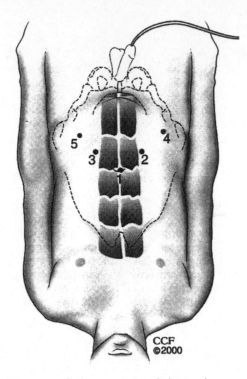

Figure 11 Trocar sites for laparoscopic radial prostalectomy.
Reprinted with permission from *The Urologic Clinics of North America*, Volume 28, Number 2, May 2001, p. 424. © WB Saunders Company.

Hormone therapy

The manipulation of the disease's natural history and symptoms through the use of hormones.

Hormone therapy, through the use of pills, shots, both pills and shots, or bilateral orchiectomy, is a palliative approach to the treatment of prostate cancer. By removing or preventing the action of testosterone on the prostate cancer, these therapies shrink the prostate cancer and slow down its growth. However, they do not cure prostate cancer (see Question 75).

Various chemotherapy regimens are being evaluated to identify drugs that may be effective against prostate cancer. The ideal drug would be one that kills the prostate cancer, rather than just slowing down its growth. Recently, the Food and Drug Administration has approved the use of certain chemotherapies for

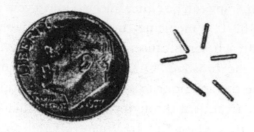

Figure 12 Actual size of I-125 seeds used for brachytherapy.
Reprinted with permission of Nycomed Amersham.

men with hormone resistant prostate cancer. Clinical trials are being performed to identify new medications and combinations of medications in hopes of identifying more effective therapies with fewer side effects (see Questions 79 and 89).

Radiation therapy is typically used as palliative treatment for patients with pain caused by bone metastases.

Intravenous (IV) medications (i.e., those administered into the veins) may also be used to treat painful bone metastases (see Question 90).

Chemotherapy is the use of powerful drugs either to kill cancer cells or interfere with their growth. Chemotherapy drugs are good at fighting cancer because they affect mostly fast-multiplying cancer cells. Some healthy cells in the body also divide quickly, such as cells that produce hair, blood, nails, and the lining of the mouth and intestinal tract. Cells in these parts of the body can be harmed by chemotherapy. Therefore, some common side effects of chemotherapy include hair loss, low white-blood–cell count, nail changes, mouth and throat irritation, nausea, and vomiting.

Radiation therapy
Use of radioactive beams or implants to kill cancer cells.

Chemotherapy
A treatment for cancer that uses powerful medications to weaken and destroy the cancer cells.

Chemotherapy can be either injected into a vein or taken by mouth. The medicine then travels throughout the body to reach some cancer cells that may have spread beyond the prostate. Often, patients who are given hormone therapy prior to chemotherapy continue their hormone treatment through the course of their chemotherapy. In studies, this treatment offered no survival benefit and helped only to reduce pain (see Question 79).

48. How do I decide which treatment is best for me?

Currently, the burden of medical decision-making falls on you, the patient, and it is our job as physicians to provide you with the information that will allow you to make the decision. When forced to make a difficult decision, we often rely on loved ones, close friends, and knowledgeable individuals to help us, but these people do not have to live with the effects of that decision. As you weigh the pros and cons of each of the various treatment options, it is very important that you think of how they will affect you. Now is the time to be very honest with yourself about what side effects you can and cannot tolerate. It is your physician's responsibility to accurately inform you of the likelihood of side effects of each of the treatment options and the remedies that are available to treat those side effects. When faced with a diagnosis of prostate cancer, the first impulse may be to get rid of the cancer at any cost. Unfortunately, once the prostate cancer has been treated and that worry quiets down, the side effects of the treatment can become more bothersome—so you should think seriously about them beforehand.

It is your physician's responsibility to accurately inform you of the likelihood of side effects of each of the treatment options and the remedies that are available to treat those side effects.

When counseling a patient, the first question that I typically ask is "Can you live with your prostate inside of you over the long term?" If the answer is no, that you would be constantly worrying about whether cancer remained in the prostate if it were left in place, then a radical prostatectomy is probably best for you. Other issues to bear in mind are the impact of incontinence and erectile dysfunction on your lifestyle. Virtually all forms of therapy can cause erectile dysfunction. If this is particularly worrisome to you, then it may be appropriate to meet with a urologist who treats erectile dysfunction to discuss the treatment options before you begin treatment for your prostate cancer. Similarly, it may be helpful to discuss the various treatments for incontinence or inability to urinate (**retention**) with your urologist or radiation oncologist before undergoing treatment. Your physician may make some treatment recommendations based on your age, medical conditions, and clinical stage of your prostate cancer. If you have questions as to why certain recommendations are being made, now is the time to ask them. Remember, no question is stupid. Your physician wants you to feel comfortable with your decision and will help you find the information that you need. There are also organizations that can provide you with information regarding treatment and side effects (see Appendix).

In an effort to help determine which therapies have the best chance of curing you of your prostate cancer, researchers have stratified prostate cancer into low-risk, intermediate-risk, and high-risk for disease progression. The treatment recommendations vary with the risk:

Retention

Difficulty in emptying the bladder of urine, may be complete, in which one is unable to void, or partial, in which urine is left in the bladder after voiding.

Low risk:

> T1c or T2a prostate cancer
>
> PSA < 10 ng/mL
>
> Gleason score < 6

Intermediate risk:

> Clinical stage T2b
>
> Gleason score 7
>
> PSA > 10 ng/mL < 20 ng/mL

High risk:

> Clinical stage T2c or higher
>
> PSA > 20 ng/mL
>
> Gleason score > 8

Low-risk patients usually do well with a single therapy such as radical prostatectomy, external beam radiation therapy, or interstitial seed therapy. High-risk patients are more likely to experience a treatment failure and combination therapy such as external beam therapy and hormonal therapy is often recommended.

49. Some of my good friends have prostate cancer and have undergone various treatments with good results. Should I have what they had?

It is often helpful to discuss with your friends how they made their final treatment decisions. They may be able to help you develop a list of questions and concerns to address with your doctor(s). Remember, however, that everyone is different and what may be appropriate for your friend may not be appropriate for you. Your Gleason score, PSA, volume of cancer, and overall health status may be different from those of your friends. Your friend may not be able to cope with his prostate remaining in place and may desire a radical prostatectomy at all costs; whereas you may be very concerned about urinary incontinence, and this concern may drive your decision making. Thus, the ultimate decision should be yours.

50. How do I select my urologist, radiation oncologist, and/or oncologist?

Cliff's comment:

My first urologist, the individual who performed my prostate biopsies, thoroughly explained the three options of treatment to me: radiation, seeds, or radical prostatectomy. However, his presentation was abrupt, showed no compassion, and sounded like a recited speech. I had done some reading on prostate cancer and asked him some questions. When I tried to discuss his qualifications and his success with preserving erectile function, his response was that his results are as good as any other doctors in the area and that if I wanted better to go to Johns Hopkins. Then he bluntly said that I should just assume that I would be impotent after the surgery—he WASN'T FOR ME! The urologist that I ultimately chose to perform my surgery was patient, sympathetic to my situation and feelings, and discussed with me the issue of potency and his success rates with the nerve-sparing radical prostatectomy. He indicated that given my Gleason score, PSA, and biopsy results, he would try to spare one set of nerves in the hope of preserving my erectile function. HE WAS THE ONE FOR ME!

As discussed in Question 46, it is common for prostate cancer patients to be treated by a multidisciplinary team of physicians and other healthcare providers. This team system, in which each clinician provides care in his or

When choosing a urologist for your prostate biopsies (and subsequent management if the biopsies are positive), you should consider a urologist who deals with prostate cancer on a regular basis.

Complication

An undesirable result of a treatment, surgery, or medication.

her area of medical expertise, has become a standard approach in modern cancer treatment.

If your primary care provider is performing your prostate cancer screening and detects an abnormality in your PSA and/or rectal examination, he or she may refer you to a urologist or to a urology practice for further evaluation. When choosing a urologist for your prostate biopsies (and subsequent management if the biopsies are positive), you should consider a urologist who deals with prostate cancer on a regular basis. Several issues should be considered when you select a physician:

Competence. You want a capable doctor who is knowledgeable and can apply that knowledge.

Technical skills. If you are planning to have prostate cancer surgery, you want to select an individual who performs a lot of radical prostatectomies. The urologist should know his or her own complication rate (a **complication** is an undesirable result of a treatment) and success rate and should feel comfortable discussing these with you. The old dictum "practice makes perfect" holds true to some extent.

Compassion. Cancer is a scary word and disease no matter how you look at it. You want a physician who understands this and is willing to take the time to help you make your management decision so that you will feel comfortable with your decision.

Approachability. As you go through the decision-making process, you want to be able to ask questions of your physician and have these questions answered in a timely manner. Delays in diagnosis and treatment only add to your anxiety.

Communication. You should expect that the team of physicians and others who are managing your case will communicate appropriately and effectively with one another as well as directly with you.

The same concepts apply in your choice of an **oncologist** (a medical specialist who is trained to evaluate and treat cancer) or **radiation oncologist** (a physician who treats cancer through the use of radiation therapy). Friends who have prostate cancer may also be able to assist you with the identification of a urologist, oncologist, or radiation oncologist who specializes in the treatment of prostate cancer.

Oncologist

A medical specialist who is trained to evaluate and treat cancer.

Radiation oncologist

A physician who treats cancer through the use of radiation therapy.

51. Should I get a second opinion?

Cliff's comment:

I think a second opinion is imperative if you have any doubt in your mind. Remember, it is your life and you want the best advice.

The decision of how best to treat your prostate cancer is a big one. You may feel very comfortable with the information that you have been given by your urologist/radiation oncologist/oncologist and you may be comfortable making an educated decision. If you do not feel that you have received enough information or you are concerned about the treatment recommendations that your urologist/radiation oncologist/oncologist is making, then it is appropriate to seek a second opinion. With all forms of therapy, it is important to ensure that those at the location where you will be receiving treatment are experienced with the form of therapy that you are selecting. It is not unreasonable to ask the urologist or radiation oncologist/oncologist what his or her or the institution's success, failure, and complication rates are. It is easy for the doctor to quote the results of large studies that show a course of treatment to be effective and safe, but what is important to you are the results of your local team. If you are concerned because of lack of information regarding these results, it may also be appropriate to seek a second opinion. Some patients are afraid to seek second opinions because they are worried that their doctor will be offended, but most physicians understand the difficult decisions that you have to make and want you to feel as comfortable as you can with your decision. In fact, many help arrange for copies of your pathology reports, clinic notes, lab tests, and X-ray results to be forwarded to the doctor you are seeing for a second opinion.

52. What is a radical prostatectomy? What are the risks and complications of radical prostatectomy?

Radical prostatectomy is the surgical procedure whereby the entire prostate is removed, as well as the seminal vesicles, the section of the urethra that passes through the prostate, the ends of the vas deferens, and a portion of the bladder neck. After the prostate and surrounding structures are removed, the bladder is then reattached to the remaining urethra. A **catheter**, which is a hollow tube, is placed through the penis into the bladder before the stitches that attach the bladder to the urethra are tied down. The catheter allows urine to drain while the bladder and urethra heal together. Because some mild bleeding, lymph drainage, and urine drainage may occur, a small drain is often placed through the skin of the abdomen into the pelvis. This drain is removed when the fluid output decreases. At the time of radical prostatectomy, depending on the approach used, the pelvic lymph nodes, which

Catheter

A hollow tube that allows for fluid drainage from or injection into an area.

are a common location of prostate cancer metastases, may also be removed (see Question 44). A radical prostatectomy may be performed via three different approaches. The most common is the retropubic approach, in which an incision is made that extends from the umbilicus (belly button) to the symphysis pubis (pubic bone) (Figure 9). The radical prostatectomy may also be performed laparoscopically through several small incisions made in various locations in the abdomen (Figure 11), or through a perineal approach, with the incision being made in the area between the scrotum and the anus (Figure 10). More recently, the radical prostatectomy may be performed with the use of a robot, robotic-assisted radical prostatectomy.

Radical prostatectomy differs from a TURP and an open suprapubic prostatectomy in that the entire prostate is removed in a radical prostatectomy. Therefore, unlike TURP and open suprapubic prostatectomy, the PSA should decrease to an undetectable level within a month or so after the procedure if no prostate cancer cells are present.

The decision as to what approach will be used for a radical prostatectomy depends on your urologist's preference and skills, your body characteristics, and whether a pelvic lymph node dissection is planned.

An advantage of the retropubic approach is that it allows for easy access to the pelvic lymph nodes so that a pelvic lymph node dissection can be performed easily at the same time. In addition, the blood vessels and nerves that control your potency are visualized easily. A disadvantage of this procedure is the abdominal incision, which may lead to a longer recovery time and increased discomfort and a higher blood loss compared to laparoscopic and robotic-assisted radical prostatectomy.

Radical prostatectomy is the surgical procedure whereby the entire prostate is removed, as well as the seminal vesicles, the section of the urethra that passes through the prostate, the ends of the vas deferens, and a portion of the bladder neck.

Perineal prostatectomy

Removal of the entire prostate, seminal vesicles, and part of the vas deferens through an incision made in the perineum.

Laparoscopic radical prostatectomy

Removal of the entire prostate, seminal vesicles, and part of the vas deferens via the laparoscope.

Laparoscopic radical prostatectomy is a procedure that has the advantages of the retropubic approach, but because there are several small abdominal incisions as opposed to the longer midline incision, the discomfort is less and the recovery is quicker with this approach.

The **perineal prostatectomy** does not involve an abdominal incision and is reported to be less uncomfortable and the recovery period shorter. The perineal approach allows for good visualization of the outlet of the bladder and the urethra for sewing the two together; however, the nerves that control potency are not seen as easily as with the retropubic approach. Another disadvantage of this procedure is that it does not allow for removal of the pelvic lymph nodes through the perineal incision and would require an additional incision for the pelvic lymph node dissection. This procedure is best suited for overweight men, for whom the retropubic approach is more difficult.

Laparoscopic radical prostatectomy is a procedure that has the advantages of the retropubic approach, but because there are several small abdominal incisions as opposed to the longer midline incision, the discomfort is less and the recovery is quicker with this approach. The disadvantage of this procedure is that it is relatively new, requires a surgeon skilled in laparoscopy (surgery performed through small incisions with visualization provided by a small telescope instrument and fine instruments that fit through the small incisions), and currently appears to be taking longer to perform than a retropubic prostatectomy. The outcomes of laparoscopic prostatectomy, i.e., urinary incontinence, erectile function and positive margin (cancer cells at the edge of the specimen) rates are similar to open surgery.

Robotic-assisted prostatectomy is the newest form of minimally invasive surgery for prostate cancer. The procedure is performed using a 3-armed robot. The robot is controlled by the surgeon, who sits at a specialized desk and controls movement of the robot's arms. Advantages of robotic-assisted prostatectomy are its ease of use compared to laparoscopy and the surgery tends to be quicker as compared to laparoscopy. In addition, the arms of the robot have movements similar to a human arm/hand/wrist, but the tremors that may be present with human movements are controlled. A disadvantage of the robot is the expense of the robot and not all hospitals can afford to purchase a robot. The outcomes with the robot are similar to those of **laparoscopic** and open radical prostatectomy; however, long-term outcomes are not available for the robot and are limited for laparoscopy. (**Figure 13**)

All surgical procedures have risks, and the common ones are infection, bleeding, pain, and anesthetic complications. Larger surgical procedures, which involve lengthier operative times and decreased postoperative mobility, have the risk of blood clots in the legs (deep venous thrombosis), pulmonary embolus, pneumonia, and stress-related stomach ulcers. Complications of radical prostatectomy include **hernia** (a weakening in the muscle that leads to a bulge), significant bleeding requiring blood transfusion, infection, anesthetic-related complications, impotence, urinary incontinence, bladder neck contracture, deep venous thrombosis, rectal injury, and death.

Robotic-assisted radical prostatectomy

A radical prostatectomy performed with the assistance of a robot.

Laparoscopy

Surgery performed through small incisions with visualization provided by a small fiberoptic instrument and fine instruments that fit through the small incisions.

Hernia

A weakening in the muscle that leads to a bulge, often in the groin.

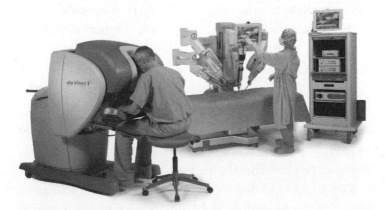

Figure 13 The da Vinci surgical system.
© 2008 Intuitive Surgical, Inc.

Bleeding

There are several large blood vessels in the pelvis and around the prostate, including the dorsal vein, which lies on top of the prostate. In order to remove the prostate, this large vein must be tied off and cut, which could cause significant and rapid bleeding. In most cases, the blood loss is less than one pint (**unit**) of blood, but in about 5% to 10% of cases, a blood transfusion is required. The amount of blood loss tends to be lower with both laparoscopic and robotic-assisted radical prostatectomies compared to open radical retropubic prostatectomy. In an attempt to decrease the need for blood transfusion, some urologists use a device called a cell saver, which takes blood that you are losing during the surgery, processes it, and returns it back to you. Thus, the blood that you get is your own. Another way to minimize the need for donor blood is to bank your own blood (autologous donation) before the surgery. Depending on your blood count and the time available before the surgery, you can donate 1 or 2 units of blood ahead of time. The advantage of autologous blood donation is that if you should require a blood transfusion, you can receive your own blood. The disadvantages of autologous blood donation, both theoretical and real, are that (1) you often begin with a lower than normal blood count (anemic), which may affect your energy level before surgery; (2) there is the rare possibility that the blood was mislabeled and that you will not receive your own blood; and (3) in the event that you do not experience significant bleeding, you do not automatically get your blood back, and you may end up being anemic and fatigued until your body replaces the blood cells. In fact, only about 21% of the autologous blood donated is actually used. In addition, if you do not need your blood, it cannot be given to another individual in need of blood. Because the risk of needing a blood transfusion is low, most people are not

Unit

Term referring to a pint of blood.

pursuing autologous blood donation, and if you do experience significant bleeding and require a transfusion of blood from the blood bank, the risk of getting acquired immunodeficiency syndrome (AIDS) or hepatitis is low because of our advanced ability to check blood donors for these diseases.

Some people ask if they could have a family member donate blood for their use if needed. This can be done, but the family member's blood type must match yours. In addition, there is actually a higher risk of hepatitis and AIDS with family/friend-directed donation than from the general population of blood donors who donate blood regularly and are screened for these diseases regularly.

Infection

Several different types of infections can occur with this surgery. A skin infection (cellulitis) may occur at the incision, an abscess (a collection of pus) may occur under the skin or deep in the pelvis, or a urinary tract infection may occur. A skin infection at the incision typically presents with redness, swelling, tenderness, and occasionally, drainage at the incision. In the absence of pus, this usually can be treated successfully with oral antibiotics; rarely, intravenous antibiotics are indicated.

Abscesses are collections of pus and may occur just under the skin or deeper in the pelvis and require drainage. More superficial abscesses can be treated by opening the incision, draining the pus, and packing the wound with sterile gauze; the packing is continued until the area heals. If the abscess is in the pelvis, it can often be treated by placing a drain through the skin into the abscess and draining the pus. This is often done under X-ray guidance by an interventional radiologist.

Urinary tract infections result from the catheter, which drains the bladder during the healing process. The risk of a urinary tract infection increases with the number of days that the catheter is in place. Because most urologists leave the catheter in for 1 to 2 weeks after the surgery, your urologist may have you drop a urine sample off at the lab 2 to 3 days before the catheter is removed so that they can detect whether any bacteria is present and if so, treat them to prevent an infection after the catheter has been removed. Signs of a urinary tract infection include frequent urination, urgency and discomfort with urination, and sometimes a low-grade fever.

Anesthetic Complications

Most patients undergo **general anesthesia** (anesthesia involving total loss of consciousness) for their radical prostatectomy; however, the procedure may be performed under spinal anesthesia. **Epidural anesthesia** is used frequently to improve postoperative pain control and decrease intraoperative anesthetic requirements. The most commonly encountered side effects of general anesthesia are scratchy throat, nausea, and vomiting, but significant anesthetic complications are rare. With epidural catheters, potential side effects include lowering of the blood pressure and muscle blocks, which may affect movement of a leg.

Impotence

Impotence, or **erectile dysfunction**, is unfortunately a commonly identified risk of radical prostatectomy. The nerves that supply the penis and that are involved in the erectile process lie along each side of the prostate and the urethra. They may be taken deliberately by the surgeon (non–nerve-sparing radical prostatectomy), or they may be injured permanently or transiently. When

General anesthesia

Anesthesia which involves total loss of consciousness.

Epidural anesthesia

A special type of anesthesia whereby pain medications are placed through a catheter in the back, into the fluid that surrounds the spinal cord.

Erectile dysfunction

The inability to achieve and/or maintain an erection satisfactory for the completion of sexual performance.

The most commonly encountered side effects of general anesthesia are scratchy throat, nausea, and vomiting, but significant anesthetic complications are rare.

the surgeon tries to avoid injury to the nerves, this is called a nerve-sparing prostatectomy. The decision to try to spare one or both nerve bundles varies with your surgeon's expertise, your Gleason score, your PSA level, and the volume (amount) of tumor on the biopsies. The incidence of postoperative erectile dysfunction may be as low as 25% in men younger than 60 who undergo bilateral nerve-sparing radical prostatectomy, or it may be as high as 62% in men older than 70 who undergo unilateral nerve-sparing radical prostatectomy. Many factors can affect your erectile function after surgery, including your erectile function before surgery, your age, your pathological tumor stage, and the extent of preservation of the nerves. Erectile dysfunction after radical prostatectomy may resolve over the first year or two after surgery. During that time and if the trouble persists, you may seek treatment for it (see Question 91). After a radical prostatectomy, you have no ejaculate because the sources of the fluid are either removed (prostate and seminal vesicles) or tied off (the vas deferens). However, you may still experience climax (reach an orgasm).

Urinary Incontinence

Urinary incontinence is another risk of radical prostatectomy.

Cliff's comment:

I feared this risk the most. I remember getting the diapers and pads the day that I had my catheter removed—my God, I thought, I am 60 years old and I'm going to be wearing diapers. Needless to say, my wife had no sympathy when I moaned about the possibility of having to wear a pad. I was lucky, however; I had two small "spills" at night and that was it for my incontinence. I discarded all of those diapers and pads within a week.

Many factors can affect your erectile function after surgery, including your erectile function before surgery, your age, your pathological tumor stage, and the extent of preservation of the nerves.

Urinary incontinence

The unintentional loss of urine.

Incontinence may vary from none to persistent incontinence, such that every time you move you leak urine. The more common type of incontinence is stress-related incontinence, which is leakage that occurs when you increase the pressure in your abdomen, such as when you bear down, pick up something heavy, laugh, or cough. The incidence of incontinence varies from 1% to 58%, and one of the reasons for the wide range in the reported incidence of incontinence is that the definition of incontinence varies. If one considers any leakage that occurs to be incontinence, then the incidence would be higher than if incontinence were defined as leakage sufficient to change a pad a day. As with erectile dysfunction, incontinence may improve or resolve over time. Risks for incontinence after surgery include prior pelvic irradiation and older age. Many options are available for the treatment of urinary incontinence after radical prostatectomy (see Question 92).

Bladder Neck Contracture

Bladder neck contracture

Scar tissue at the bladder neck that causes narrowing.

A **bladder neck contracture** is scar tissue that develops in the area where the bladder and urethra are sewn together. This problem occurs in about 1 in every 20 to 30 prostatectomies. The signs and symptoms of a bladder neck contracture include decreased force of stream and straining (pushing) to urinate. The bladder neck contracture is identified during an office cystoscopy, in which a **cystoscope**, a telescope-like instrument, is passed through the urethra up to the bladder neck and the narrowed area is visualized. If the opening is very small, a small wire can be passed through it and the area dilated (stretched open) using some metal or plastic dilators in the office. Before the procedure, the urethra is numbed with lidocaine jelly to decrease discomfort. Usually, once the bladder neck is dilated, it remains open;

Cystoscope

A telescope-like instrument that allows one to examine the urethra and inside of the bladder.

however, in a small number of men, a repeat dilation or an incision into the scar under anesthesia is needed. A complication of treatment for bladder neck contracture is urinary incontinence.

Deep Venous Thrombosis

A **deep venous thrombosis (DVT)** is a blood clot that develops in the veins in the leg or the pelvis. People with cancer and those who are sedentary are at increased risk for such blood clots. During surgery and your initial postoperative period, you are not moving around much and are at increased risk for forming blood clots. Thromboembolic (TED) hose and Venodynes (pneumatic sequential stockings that inflate and deflate to keep blood flowing) are often used during this period to decrease the risk of forming such blood clots. DVTs may cause swelling of the leg, which often resolves when the blood clot dissolves. A more serious risk posed by a DVT is that a piece of the clot could break off and travel to the heart and lungs; this is called a pulmonary embolus. A pulmonary embolus can be life threatening if the fragment is large enough to block off blood flow to the lung. Although rare, pulmonary emboli are one of the causes of sudden death after surgery and may occur days to weeks after surgery. Because the pulmonary embolus decreases blood flow to the lungs, it can cause difficulty breathing. DVTs are often treated with blood thinners to break down the clot and prevent it from getting larger. If you are at high risk (likely) for a pulmonary embolus or are not a candidate for blood thinners, a filter, which is a metal device that catches clots and prevents them from traveling to the heart and lungs, would be placed into the main vein of the body (the vena cava). In this procedure, for which you would receive local anesthesia (control of your pain in the area

Deep venous thrombosis (DVT)

The formation of a blood clot in the large deep veins, usually of the legs or in the pelvis.

involved in the surgery), a needle followed by a catheter is inserted into the main vein in the groin, the femoral vein, and the filter is passed up into the vena cava, where it is allowed to expand. Because DVTs and pulmonary emboli occur most commonly after discharge from the hospital, if you should develop acute swelling in your leg, pain in your calf, or shortness of breath, you must contact your doctor immediately. If you are not walking around much at home during your first week after surgery, it may be helpful to continue to wear the TED hose stockings.

Rectal Injury

The incidence of rectal injury during a radical prostatectomy is less than 2%. There is a slightly higher risk of rectal injury with the perineal approach (1.73%) than with the retropubic approach (0.68%). In most cases, if the injury is small and you have performed the bowel prep and no stool is visible, then the area can be closed and should heal. For large injuries that occur with bowels that are not well prepped, a temporary **colostomy** (the bowel is brought to the skin to drain the stool into a bag) is made to decrease the chances of stool leakage and abscess formation; the colostomy can be removed later.

Colostomy

A surgical opening between the colon (large intestine) and the skin that allows stool to drain into a collecting bag.

Miscellaneous Complications Related to the Radical Prostatectomy

The retropubic prostatectomy has a higher risk of cardiovascular, respiratory, and other medically related complications, primarily **gastrointestinal** (i.e., related to the digestive system or intestines), such as slow return of bowel function, than the perineal approach. The perineal approach has a higher risk of miscellaneous surgical complications, such as rectal injury and postoperative infections. The perineal approach may also be

Gastrointestinal (GI)

Related to the digestive system and/or the intestines.

associated with an increased risk of incontinence of stool. The incidence of complications and **mortality** (death) increases with patient age at the time of surgery.

Mortality
Death related to disease or treatment.

Death

The mortality rate associated with radical prostatectomy is less than 0.1%.

53. What is a nerve-sparing radical prostatectomy?

The nerves responsible for erectile function run along each side of the prostate and along each side of the ure-thra before passing out of the pelvis into the penis. These nerves travel along with blood vessels, and the group is called the "neurovascular bundle," which lies outside of the prostate capsule. These nerves are not responsible for control of urine—only erectile function. During a **nerve-sparing prostatectomy**, the urologist attempts to dissect (push aside) the neurovascular bundle from the prostate and the urethra. The surgeon may perform a bilateral nerve-sparing radical prostatectomy, in which the neurovascular bundle on each side is spared, or a unilateral nerve-sparing prostatectomy, in which one neurovascular bundle is removed with the prostate. The decision of whether or not to perform a nerve-sparing rad-ical prostatectomy depends on many issues, one of which is your erectile function. If you already have erectile dys-function, then sparing the nerves is not an issue. Other considerations include the amount of tumor present in your biopsy specimen, the location of the tumor (whether it is in both sides of the prostate), and the Gleason score. Remember that a radical prostatectomy is a cancer opera-tion, and the goal of the procedure is to try to remove all of the cancer. Therefore, if you are at high risk for having

Nerve-sparing
With regard to pros-tate cancer, it is the attempt to not dam-age or remove the nerves that lie on either side of the prostate gland that are in part responsi-ble for normal erec-tions. Injury to the nerves can cause erectile dysfunction.

87

cancer at the edge of the prostate, it is better to remove the neurovascular bundle(s) and surrounding tissue on that side in hopes of removing all of the cancer. A bilateral nerve-sparing radical prostatectomy does not guarantee that you will have normal erectile function after the surgery. You should consider this fact and decide before surgery how much of an impact postoperative erectile dysfunction would have on your life.

54. Who is a candidate for radical prostatectomy?

The ideal candidate for a radical prostatectomy is a man who is believed to have prostate cancer that is confined to the prostate gland, is healthy enough to withstand the general anesthesia and the surgical procedure, and is expected to live for at least an additional 7 to 10 years so that he will benefit from the surgery.

The ideal candidate for a radical prostatectomy is a man who is believed to have prostate cancer that is confined to the prostate gland, is healthy enough to withstand the general anesthesia and the surgical procedure, and is expected to live for at least an additional 7 to 10 years so that he will benefit from the surgery. It is difficult to determine who really has organ-confined disease, or cancer that is apparently confined to the prostate. Tables may help estimate the risks of having tumor outside of the prostate, but these are only part of the decision-making process. Approximately 20% to 60% of men undergoing radical prostatectomy have a higher stage of prostate cancer when the pathologist reviews the surgical specimen.

Just because you are a candidate for a radical prostatectomy does not mean that this is the best form of treatment for you. You must look carefully at your lifestyle, the risks of the surgery, and what is most important to you regarding your quality of life before making a decision. If, for example, the possibility of urinary incontinence would be devastating to you, then maybe surgery is not the best therapy for you. On the other hand, if the idea of leaving your prostate in place will constantly worry you, then perhaps surgery is best for you.

55. *How does one prepare for radical prostatectomy?*

Cliff's comment:

As you prepare for surgery and try to optimize your physical health by eating right, resting, and getting exercise, it is also important to make sure that you are able to cope mentally with all of the stress caused by the diagnosis and treatment of a cancer. I knew I was anxious about my surgery, but I was never able to correlate the significance of that until after the surgery, when I realized that I had increased the dose of my blood pressure medications significantly in the month before surgery. If you find that you are having trouble emotionally preparing for surgery, talk with your doctor, family, or friends. They may be able to help alleviate your anxieties or refer you to another individual, such as a therapist, psychologist, or psychiatrist.

In preparation for surgery, you will undergo a history and physical examination, some blood tests, and often a chest X-ray study and electrocardiogram. These assessments are performed to make sure that you are healthy enough for surgery and to rule out any medical problems that may increase your risk of complications after surgery. You should eat a healthy diet and continue to exercise before the surgery. Starting about 10 days before surgery, you should not take any medications that contain aspirin or nonsteroidal anti-inflammatory drugs, because they might increase your risk of bleeding during the surgery. Many over-the-counter medications contain one of these, and if you are unsure about whether yours does, you should consult a pharmacist. If you were prescribed aspirin because of heart disease, then you should speak to your primary care doctor or heart doctor before stopping the aspirin.

Bowel prep

Cleansing (and sterilization) of the intestines before abdominal surgery.

Your urologist may give you a **bowel preparation** to clean out the lower intestines. This may involve drinking a special fluid to clean your bowels out or using an enema. You may also be asked to have a clear liquid diet the day before surgery.

56. What is the hospital course like?

Cliff's comment:

I envisioned staying in the hospital 2 to 3 days after my surgery, staying locally until the catheter was removed, and then returning home. Although my biggest fear, that of not waking up after the surgery, did not occur, I did have a rocky postoperative course and remained in the hospital for about two weeks and had the catheter in place longer. I found the catheter to be most annoying initially. I had a visiting nurse who taught me how to use the drainage bags, and I got used to the catheter, but I must admit, the day of the catheter removal was a glorious day—the ability to urinate again on my own and to control urination again felt wonderful. Thank God for those small pleasures!

Typically, you are admitted to the hospital the day of your surgery, and you usually stay in the hospital 2 to 3 nights (inpatient), including the night of your surgery for the radical retropubic prostatectomy.

Typically, you are admitted to the hospital the day of your surgery, and you usually stay in the hospital 2 to 3 nights (inpatient), including the night of your surgery for the radical retropubic prostatectomy. Men undergoing laparoscopic and robotic-assisted radical prostatectomies may go home as soon as the day after surgery and tend to be fully recovered more quickly than those who undergo the traditional radical retropubic prostatectomy. Most men go from the recovery room to a regular hospital room, with very few needing a bed in the intensive care unit (ICU).

An epidural catheter, which is a small catheter placed through the lower back into the space around the spinal cord at the time of your surgery, may be used for postoperative pain control. Pain medications can be given through the catheter to numb the nerves so that you do not feel pain. Another way to control postoperative pain is with a patient-controlled analgesia pump, which is an intravenous form of pain medication controlled by a small button that you press when you want pain medication. Once you are tolerating liquids, oral pain medications may be used; some physicians use narcotics, whereas others use strong anti-inflammatories.

The nurses will teach you how to use the urinary drainage bags and will assist you with getting into and out of bed. You will go home when you are comfortable while taking oral pain medications and your bowels are working. You will be discharged with a **Foley catheter,** which drains the urine and will be in place 7 days to 2 weeks to allow the area where the bladder has been reattached to the urethra to heal. At home, you can resume your regular diet and slowly increase your activity level. Depending on the approach used, your full recovery may take up to one month.

Foley catheter

A latex or silicone catheter that drains urine from the bladder.

When your catheter is removed, you will be taught Kegel exercises (pelvic muscle strengthening exercises), which will help you control your urine. Most individuals regain nearly all or full control of their urine by one month after the catheter is removed. Your PSA level will be checked 4 to 6 weeks after surgery to make sure that it has decreased to an undetectable level.

57. What is the success rate of radical prostatectomy?

Cliff's comment:

It has been 2 ½ years since my radical prostatectomy, and I feel great. I am doing all of the things that I had done before the surgery and more. So far, my PSA has remained undetectable, and it is very reassuring to hear this at my urology clinic visits.

In general, more than 70% of properly selected cases (i.e., men who are believed to have prostate cancer that is clinically confined to the prostate) remain free of tumor for more than 7 to 10 years. If one has a T2 tumor (see Question 42), the probability of remaining free from PSA elevation can be as high as 90% if there were no **positive margins** (tumor at the edge of the specimen). However, it is hard to predict before surgery who is the best candidate for surgery because 30% to 40% of patients are diagnosed with a higher stage or grade of cancer when the surgical specimen is reviewed by the pathologist. Positive surgical margins are found in 14% to 41% of men undergoing radical prostatectomy, and in those men with positive margins, there is an almost 50% chance that the PSA will increase within 5 years after surgery. This varies with the amount of tumor at the margin and the location of the positive margin. Your urologist would discuss whether additional therapy is indicated if the margin is positive. Men with negative margins have only an 18% chance of the PSA rising at 5 years after surgery. Initially after surgery, you will have your PSA level checked on an every-3-month basis. Depending on the lab that your physician uses, a PSA level < 0.1 ng/mL or a PSA level < 0.02 ng/mL may be reported as undetectable. The numbers vary because the **sensitivity** in PSA testing varies from lab to lab. If

Positive margin

The presence of cancer cells at the cut edge of tissue removed during surgery: A positive margin indicates that there may be cancer cells remaining in the body.

Sensitivity

The probability that a diagnostic test can correctly identify the presence of a particular disease.

the PSA remains undetectable after one year, then your urologist may order PSA testing on an every-6-month basis for about one year, after which you will continue with yearly PSA tests. Depending on your pathology report and your urologist's preference, you may also have a digital rectal examination at the time of your PSA.

Cliff's comment:

The first PSA test after surgery is the most suspenseful. Even though your urologist may tell you that your pathology specimen from surgery looks good and that there are no cancer cells at the margins (the edges of the tissue), you are still anxious to hear what the PSA is. You want it to be undetectable—you want it to indicate that the cancer has been "caught" and removed. You get your blood drawn and then you wait to meet with your urologist or for the phone call regarding your results. I remember how happy I felt when I got my first PSA report after the surgery. Now, 2½ years later, I am still slightly anxious when I have my PSA drawn, although as each year goes by the anxiety is decreasing. With each good PSA result, I start to believe that "they've gotten it all." I realize that it will be an additional seven more years before I can technically say I am cured, but each year that goes by that I am healthy and the PSA remains undetectable is another year enjoyed and another year closer to that goal.

58. What is brachytherapy/interstitial seed therapy? What are the side effects and complications of interstitial seeds or brachytherapy?

Brachytherapy derives from the Greek word "brachy," which means near to. Brachytherapy is a technique in which either permanent radioactive seeds or temporary needles are placed directly into the prostate gland

(**Figures** 13 and **14**). This form of therapy started in the early 1900s and then had a resurgence in the 1970s but was abandoned because of difficulties with accurate seed placement. With the development of transrectal ultrasound, the use of C-arm fluoroscopy, and more recently, the use of three-dimensional computerized treatment planning and postoperative CT-based dosimetry, the procedure has become technically easier and more precise. As a result, it is gaining in popularity.

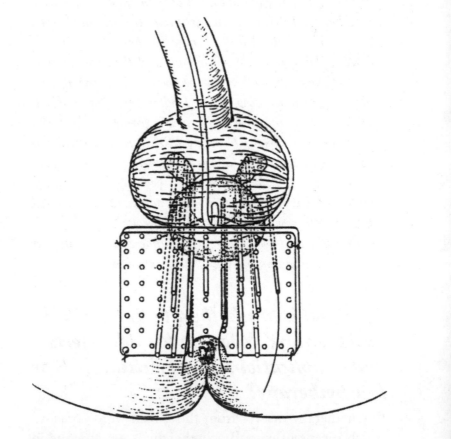

Figure 14 Template used to guide interstitial seed placement.
Reprinted with permission with Bagshaw M, Kaplan ID, Cox RC, *Cancer* 1993; 71 (suppl): 939–952. Copyright © 1993, American Cancer Society. Reprinted with permission of Wiley-Liss, Inc., a subsidary of John Wiley & Sons, Inc.

Before the seeds are placed, either a transrectal ultrasound or a CT scan of the prostate is performed to assess the prostate volume. This helps determine needle placement and seed positioning within the needle. Typically, the target volume includes the original prostate volume plus 2-mm margins laterally and anterior to the prostate gland, as well as additional 5-mm margins at the top and bottom of the prostate. This measurement is done to try to ensure that the prostatic capsule is included in the treatment. No additional margins are added posteriorly to prevent injury to the rectum. It is also important to limit the dose received by the urethra to prevent urethral irritation. The radiation dose typically ranges from 125 Gy to 144 Gy.

The most commonly encountered side effects of interstitial seed therapy include voiding troubles related to bladder outlet obstruction, urinary incontinence, and rectal ulceration and bleeding. In addition, in some patients a benign increase in the PSA may occur after interstitial seed therapy. Urinary symptoms occur earlier with palladium because it releases high energy earlier than iodine. Individuals may develop urinary **frequency** (frequent urination), dysuria, or urinary retention. Urinary symptoms, if they are not associated with urinary retention, are often treated with nonsteroidal anti-inflammatories and an alpha-blocker and often resolve over 1 to 4 months, but may persist for 12 to 18 months.

Frequency

A term used to describe the need to urinate often.

Bladder Outlet Obstruction

Trouble urinating after interstitial seed therapy occurs in 7% to 25% of cases, possibly as a result of blood clots in the bladder or swelling of the prostate. About 10% of men will experience acute urinary retention, the inability to urinate on their own, requiring temporary placement of a Foley catheter. If the cause is blood clots, then the clots are washed out of the bladder and a Foley catheter may be left in place for a few days. If the problems with voiding are believed to be caused by prostate swelling, then a catheter may be left in place for a short period of time, and your doctor may want you to try some medications, including an alpha-blocker or an anti-inflammatory. If you are not able to void for awhile, then a suprapubic tube or clean intermittent **catheterization** may be easier for you. A suprapubic tube is a catheter that is placed through the skin of the lower abdomen into the bladder to drain the urine. It remains in place until you can urinate on your own. It has the advantages of being able to be changed on a monthly basis in your urologist's office, and it does not cause urethral irritation like a Foley catheter.

Clean intermittent catheterization (CIC)

The placement of a catheter into the bladder to drain urine and the removal after the urine is drained at defined intervals throughout the day to allow for bladder emptying. It may also be performed to maintain patency after treatment of a bladder neck contracture or urethral stricture.

Clean intermittent catheterization involves placing a catheter through the penis into the bladder to drain the bladder on a regular schedule (usually every 4 to 6 hours) throughout the day. The advantages of clean intermittent catheterization are that it allows you to know when you are able to void on your own, it minimizes bladder and urethral irritation, and it has less risk of infections and bladder stones over the long term. Although it is discouraging to be unable to urinate after the procedure, it is important to allow time to pass and see whether the problem will resolve. A TURP should be delayed to give you a sufficient trial because of the increased risk of urinary incontinence.

Urinary Incontinence

Urinary incontinence is uncommon in men undergoing interstitial seed therapy. In men who have not had a prior TURP (transurethral resection of the prostate), incontinence occurs in less than 1%. In men who have had a prior TURP, the risk of incontinence is 25% and is up to 40% if more than one TURP has been performed.

Rectal Ulceration/Bleeding

Rectal irritation does not occur as commonly as urinary symptoms and tends to improve quicker than urinary symptoms. Less than 5% of patients will have a rectal ulcer or rectal bleeding, which occurs as a result of irritation of the rectal lining. It may be associated with pain, rectal spasms, and the feeling that one needs to have a bowel movement. This condition can be treated with several topical medications and a low-roughage diet.

PSA "Bounce" or "Blip"

This occurs when the PSA increases on two consecutive blood draws and then decreases and remains low without rising again. The cause of this phenomenon is not known. It occurs in about one third of men treated with interstitial seeds and typically occurs around 9 to 24 months after the treatment. It may or may not be accompanied by symptoms of prostate inflammation; if such symptoms are present, then treatment for prostatitis may decrease the symptoms and the PSA level.

Urethral Stricture

This narrowing of the urethra is related to the development of scar tissue; it is uncommon after interstitial seeds, ocurring in 5–12% of men, and tends to develop later. It may present with a change in the force of stream or the need to strain to void. A stricture is identified by cystoscopy in the doctor's office. Treatment of the stricture depends on the location and the extent of the stricture; it may require a simple office dilation or an incision under anesthesia.

The advantages of clean intermittent catheterization are that it allows you to know when you are able to void on your own, it minimizes bladder and urethral irritation, and it has less risk of infections and bladder stones over the long term.

Erectile Dysfunction

This condition may occur in as many as 40% to 60% of men who undergo interstitial seed therapy. Unlike radical prostatectomy, the erectile dysfunction tends to occur a year or more after the procedure and not right away. There is an increased risk of post seed therapy erectile dysfunction in older men and in those receiving hormone therapy. Erectile dysfunction after interstitial seed therapy responds well to a variety of treatment options (see Question 91).

59. Who is a candidate for interstitial seed therapy?

Similar to radical prostatectomy, the goal of interstitial therapy is to cure one of prostate cancer. With this in mind, the candidate should have a life expectancy of more than 7 to 10 years and no underlying illness that would contraindicate the procedure such that he will not benefit from a cure. Men with significant obstructive voiding symptoms and/or prostate volumes greater than 60 mL are at increased risk for voiding troubles and urinary retention after the procedure. Men who have undergone a prior TURP are at increased risk for urinary incontinence after brachytherapy. Men with clinically localized prostate cancer of low to intermediate risk are candidates for interstitial seed therapy. Men with high-risk prostate cancer (PSA > 20.0 ng/mL, Gleason score > 8, or stage T3a prostate cancer) should not be treated with interstitial seed therapy alone. Depending on your risk, hormonal therapy may be used in addition to interstitial seed therapy.

60. What happens the day of the procedure and what can I expect?

Your physician will give you instructions regarding your diet for the day or two before the procedure. You may be asked to have a clear liquid diet the day before the procedure and to use an enema to clean out stool from the rectum the evening before the procedure. As with any surgical procedure, you will be instructed not to eat or drink after midnight the evening before surgery. You may take your medications with a sip of water. The brachytherapy procedure is performed under anesthesia, either spinal or general. After adequate anesthesia has been obtained, you are placed in a dorsal lithotomy position. You are lying on your back, with your legs bent, elevated, and separated to allow access to the perineum and rectum. A Foley catheter is placed through the urethra into the bladder, and a small amount of contrast material (X-ray dye) is placed into the balloon of the catheter so that the balloon can be visualized under **fluoroscopy**, which involves the use of a fluoroscope, a radiologic device used for examining deep structures by means of X-rays. The catheter allows the doctor to identify where the bladder outlet is. The **bladder outlet** is the first part of the natural channel through which urine passes when it leaves the bladder. The prostate sits right below the outlet.

A repeat transrectal ultrasound is performed to measure the volume of the prostate again and to determine the number of needles and corresponding radioactive seeds, the isotope and the isotope strength necessary for the procedure. The seeds may be placed into the prostate through a variety of techniques including fluoroscopic guidance, ultrasound guidance or via the use of MRI. At the end of the procedure the catheter is removed, and a cystoscopy (a look into the bladder with a telescope-like

Fluoroscopy

Use of a fluoroscope, a radiologic device that is used for examining deep structures by means of X-rays.

Bladder outlet

The first part of the natural channel through which urine passes when it leaves the bladder.

device) may be performed to make sure that no seeds are in the bladder or urethra. If seeds are found in the bladder or urethra, they are removed.

At our institution, a catheter is placed after the cystoscopy is performed, and the patient is discharged to home with the catheter in place for 24 hours. After the procedure is completed and the patient has recovered, a CT scan is obtained and CT-based dosimetry is calculated to assess the seed placement and the dose of radiation delivered throughout the prostate.

Several terms are used to describe the dose of radiation. The D100 is the dose received by the entire prostate, the V100 is the percent of the volume of the prostate that received 100% of the prescribed dose, and the V150 is the percent of the volume of the prostate that received 150% of the prescribed dose. An acceptable seed implantation should maintain a V100 of at least 80%. Although the D100 is often below the prescribed dose as a result of the sharp decrease in the radiation dose at the edge of the implant, ideally the total dose should be about 90% of the D100 (D90).

After the procedure is performed, you may notice some swelling, black and blue coloring, or slight bleeding from the perineum (the area under the scrotum and in front of the rectum). This is related to the needle placement and usually resolves over the next few days. The area may also be tender to touch; applying ice packs intermittently to the area for the first 24 hours after the procedure helps decrease the swelling. Sitz baths, nonsteroidal anti-inflammatory drugs, and acetaminophen help reduce the discomfort. Good personal hygiene minimizes infection.

You may also notice some blood in the urine after the procedure; this is related to urethral irritation and usually resolves within 24 hours. There may also be some blood in the fluid released during **ejaculation** (the release of **semen** through the penis during orgasm), the ejaculate; in fact, the ejaculate may look brown, black, or even red after the procedure. This may seem alarming, but it is not cause for concern. The ejaculate is composed of fluid from the **testes**, the prostate, and the seminal vesicles. Thus, bleeding in the prostate or seminal vesicles that results from needle penetration may cause blood in the ejaculate, which resolves with time.

61. When can I return to work after interstitial seed therapy?

Because the procedure is minimally invasive and requires no incisions, you can typically return to work and full activity within 3 to 4 days after the procedure.

62. If I have had brachytherapy, am I a radiation risk to others?

No. Although the seeds are radioactive, you are not, and thus you are not a radiation risk to others. The seeds emit radiation, but the vast majority of the radiation is absorbed by the prostate. Intimate contact will not pass on the radiation. However, some recommend that for the first two months after seed placement, you should limit contact with small children and pregnant women.

Ejaculation
The release of semen through the penis during orgasm. After radical prostatectomy and often after a TURP, no fluid is released during orgasm.

Semen
The whitish fluid that is released during ejaculation.

Testis
One of two male reproductive organs that are located within the scrotum and produce testosterone and sperm.

You may also notice some blood in the urine after the procedure; this is related to urethral irritation and usually resolves within 24 hours.

63. Why is my radiation oncologist or urologist recommending interstitial seed therapy plus EBRT?

Interstitial seed therapy is limited in its ability to reach tissue outside of the prostate, especially the back of the prostate. The addition of EBRT may help in patients who are judged to be at high risk for disease penetrating through or outside the prostate capsule. Use of interstitial seeds alone is appropriate for patients with tumors in clinical stage T1c to T2a, a Gleason score < 6, and a PSA < 10. Patients with a Gleason score of 7 or greater, a PSA > 10, tumors in clinical stage T2b or minimal T3a, and at least four of six biopsies positive for cancer or perineural invasion on the biopsy appear to be the best served by the combination of interstitial seeds and EBRT.

64. Where can I find out who performs brachytherapy in my area, and how do I choose the appropriate individual to perform the brachytherapy?

You could call your local hospital and ask whether they have a listing of urologists/radiation oncologists that perform interstitial seed therapy in your area. You can also call a physician reference listing (800-228-0126), which provides the locations of U.S. physicians performing seed implantation. When you discuss brachytherapy with the urologist or radiation oncologist, you may wish to ask several questions, including:

(1) How long has the physician been performing brachytherapy, and how many procedures has he or she performed? (2) What is the individual's success and failure rate? (3) What is his or her complication rate? and

(4) What does the physician feel is your likelihood of success or failure and your likelihood of complications given your PSA level, Gleason grade, and overall health?

65. How am I monitored after interstitial seed placement?

Unlike with radical prostatectomy, the prostate remains in your body, and thus the PSA does not decrease to an undetectable level. In addition, it may take at least two years for the PSA to reach its lowest level (**PSA nadir**). The PSA is typically checked one month after seed placement and then every 3 to 6 months for two years thereafter if the level remains stable. After two years, the PSA is checked yearly. Failure of seed therapy is defined as a nadir of > 0.5 ng/mL to 1.0 ng/mL or three consecutive rises in the PSA level more than 3 months apart for each value. A rise in PSA may occur in as many as one third of the patients between the first and second year after the implantation. This is called a "benign PSA bump," and it appears to be related to late tissue reactions to the radiation; it does not mean that the seeds have failed or that you are at increased risk of failure. In this situation, the PSA does not continue to rise, and this is how one differentiates a PSA bump from a failure.

PSA nadir

The lowest value that the PSA reaches during a particular treatment.

66. What is the success rate of brachytherapy?

The results of prostate brachytherapy are comparable to those of radical prostatectomy for 5 to 7 years after treatment. The long-term data (i.e., the data for longer than ten years after treatment) are limited. Reported studies demonstrate success rates of 64% to 85% at ten years, with success being defined by either a PSA < 0.5 ng/mL or the absence of three consecutive rises in PSA in patients who received brachytherapy EBRT.

67. What are external-beam and conformal external-beam radiation therapy? What are the side effects of EBRT?

External-beam radiation therapy (EBRT) is the use of radiation therapy to kill or inactivate cancer cells. The total radiation dose is given in separate individual treatments, known as "fractionation." Cancer cells are most sensitive to radiation at different phases in their growth. By giving the radiation on a daily basis, the radiation oncologist hopes to catch the cancer cells in the sensitive phases of growth and also to prevent the cells from having time to recover from the radiation damage. Conformal EBRT uses CT images to help better visualize the radiation targets and the normal tissues; with three-dimensional images, the radiation oncologist can identify critical structures, such as the bladder, the rectum, and the hip bones. This allows the radiation oncologist to deliver more radiation (72–82 Gy as opposed to 66–72 Gy with standard EBRT) to the prostate tissue but decrease the amount of normal tissue that is irradiated. The advantage of conformal EBRT over EBRT is that conformal EBRT causes less rectal and urinary irritation. The construction of an immobilization device (cradle) and the placement of small, permanent tattoos ensure that you are properly positioned for the radiation treatment each day. Through the assistance of computers, the radiation oncologist can define an acceptable dose distribution to the prostate and surrounding tissues, and the computer determines the appropriate beam configuration to create this desired distribution.

The side effects of EBRT or conformal EBRT can be either acute (occurring within 90 days after EBRT) or late (occurring > 90 days after EBRT). The severity of the side effects varies with the total and the daily radiation dose, the type of treatment, the site of treatment, and the individual's tolerance. The most commonly noted side effects include changes in bowel habits, bowel bleeding, skin irritation, edema, fatigue, and urinary symptoms, including dysuria, frequency, hesitancy, and nocturia. Less commonly, swelling of the legs, scrotum, or penis may occur. Late side effects include persistence of bowel dysfunction, persistence of urinary symptoms, urinary bleeding, urethral stricture, and erectile dysfunction.

Bowel Changes

A change in bowel habits is one of the more common side effects of EBRT. Patients may develop diarrhea, abdominal cramping, the feeling of needing to have a bowel movement, rectal pain, and bleeding. Usually, if these side effects are going to occur, they do so in the second or third week of treatment.

If diarrhea is severe enough to warrant treatment, you can use medications that decrease bowel motility (i.e., medications used to treat diarrhea). Changes in dietary habits, such as eating a low-residue diet and avoiding certain foods (milk, raw vegetables, squash, gas-producing vegetables, dried fruit, fiber cereals, seeds, popcorn, nuts, chunky peanut butter, corn, and dried beans) are helpful. Drinking plenty of fluids helps prevent dehydration.

Rectal pain can be treated with warm sitz baths, hydrocortisone-containing creams, or anti-inflammatory suppositories.

Late bowel effects include persistent changes in bowel function, rectal **fistula** (a communication between the rectum and other site, e.g., the prostate or the skin), or perforation (a hole in the rectum), and bleeding. Rectal fistula and perforation are rare and often require surgical treatment.

Fistula

An abnormal passage or communication, usually between 2 internal organs, or leading from an internal organ to the surface of the body.

Skin Irritation

The tolerance of the skin to radiation depends on the dose of radiation used and the location of the skin affected. Certain areas are more sensitive than others; the perineum and the fold under the buttocks are very sensitive and may become red, flake, or drain fluid. To prevent further irritation, avoid applying soaps, deodorants, perfumes, powders, cosmetics, or lotions to the irritated skin. After you wash the area, gently blot it dry. Cotton underwear and loose-fitting clothes can help prevent further irritation. If the irritated skin is dry, topical therapies, such as petroleum jelly, lanolin, zinc oxide, corn starch, and other topical skin therapies, can be applied.

Edema

Edema of the legs, scrotum, and penis may rarely occur, but when it does, it is more common in those who have undergone prior pelvic lymph node dissection. Lower-extremity edema can be treated with supportive stockings, TED hose, and elevation of feet when sitting and lying down. Penile and scrotal edema is often difficult to treat.

Urinary Symptoms

The genitourinary symptoms of dysuria, frequency, hesitancy, and nocturia are related to changes that occur in the bladder and urethra that result from radiation exposure. The bladder may not hold much urine because of the irritation and scarring, and irritation of the bladder lining may make it more prone to bleeding. Bladder inflammation usually occurs about 3 to 5 weeks into the radiation treatments and gradually subsides about 2 to 8 weeks after the completion of radiation treatments. Urinary anesthetics and bladder relaxants may be helpful in decreasing the urinary frequency.

68. Who is a candidate for conformal EBRT?

Men who are candidates for conventional EBRT are also candidates for conformal EBRT. Similar to other curative treatments, the ideal patient has a life expectancy of 7 to 10 years. In higher-risk patients, the increased radiation dose used with conformal EBRT causes a significantly better decrease in PSA progression than the dose used in conventional EBRT. There does not appear to be a PSA progression-free survival benefit with conformal EBRT when compared with conventional EBRT in patients who have low-risk prostate cancer. Men who have a PSA level > 10 ng/mL or with a tumor that is clinical stage T3 are the most likely to benefit from the higher radiation doses that can be achieved with conformal EBRT and may benefit from combination therapy, such as hormone therapy plus EBRT. The amount of radiation and the field of radiation differ for each individual and depend on the clinical stage and the Gleason grade. Contraindications to EBRT include a history of inflammatory bowel disease, such as Crohn's disease and ulcerative colitis or a history of prior pelvic radiotherapy.

69. What does the treatment entail?

Conformal EBRT requires that you undergo a treatment planning session (simulation) that includes a CT scan. Thereafter, as with conventional EBRT, you are seen five days a week (Monday through Friday) for a short period of time to receive a treatment. The treatments last for about 6 to 7 weeks, depending on the total dose selected by your radiation oncologist. The dose received and the use of neoadjuvant or adjuvant therapy may vary with your risk factors. Hormonal therapy is often recommended for men with a Gleason score of 7 or higher or a PSA of 10 ng/ml or higher in conjunction with standard dose EBRT (about 70 cGy) or dose escalation to 78–79 cGY using 3D conformal radiation technique. In low risk patients, dose escalation appears to be beneficial. In intermediate risk patients, either a short course (about 6 months) of hormone therapy and standard dose EBRT or dose escalation is recommended. The regimen varies according to your clinical stage and whether the radiation therapy is being given as a first-line therapy or as a secondary therapy, such as for an increasing PSA after radical prostatectomy.

70. What is the success rate of EBRT or conformal EBRT?

The success rate varies with the initial PSA level. In one study, 89% to 92% of men treated with conformal EBRT whose pretreatment PSA was < 10 ng/mL showed no increase in PSA level at five years. Those with a pretreatment PSA of 10 to 19.9 ng/mL had an 82% to 86% chance of no increase in PSA level at five years, compared with a 26% to 63% chance of no increase in PSA at five years in men with a pretreatment PSA of > 20 ng/mL.

Men with T1 and T2 tumors have survival rates that are comparable to that with radical prostatectomy. In such individuals, the clinical tumor-free survival is 96% at five years and 86% at ten years.

71. What is cryotherapy/cryosurgery? What are the complications of cryotherapy?

Cryotherapy is a technique used for prostate cancer treatment that involves controlled freezing of the prostate gland. This procedure is performed under anesthesia. Transrectal ultrasound evaluation (similar to that used with your prostate biopsy) is used throughout the procedure to visualize the prostate and to monitor the position of the freezing probes, which are placed through the perineal skin (the area below the scrotum and in front of the anus) into the prostate (**Figure 15**). During the freezing, the transrectal ultrasound demonstrates an "ice ball" in the prostate. The freezing process kills both hormone-sensitive and hormone-insensitive cancer cells. Proper positioning of the probe may allow one to kill cancer cells even at the edge of the prostate, the prostate capsule.

During the freezing, a catheter is placed into the urethra, and a warming solution is run through the catheter to protect the urethra from freezing. Despite this, irritation of the urethra and/or bladder can occur and may lead to

Cryotherapy is a technique used for prostate cancer treatment that involves controlled freezing of the prostate gland.

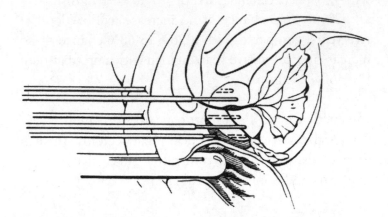

Figure 15 Placement of needles for cryoablation of the prostate.
Reprinted with permission from Clarke HS, Cyrosurgical Ablation of the Prostate. In Graham SD, Glenn JF (eds), *Glenn's Urologic Surgery* (5th Ed.), Lippincott Williams & Wilkins, 1998, p. 1101–1104.

frequency, urgency, burning, pain with urination, and blood in the urine. Similarly, irritation of the rectal wall may occur, leading to blood in the stools, rectal pain, and pain with bowel movements. Up to 80% of men undergoing cryotherapy can have troubles with erectile dysfunction, and an increased incidence occurs in men in whom attempts were made to include the prostate capsule in the freezing. Less commonly seen side effects include urethral scar formation, trouble urinating that requires a TURP (in 10% to 55% of men), and urinary incontinence. A serious complication of cryotherapy is a urethrorectal fistula, a communication between the urethra and the rectum, which can lead to leakage of urine from the rectum and urinary tract infections.

72. Who is a candidate for cryotherapy?

Currently, cryotherapy is used more commonly as a **salvage** therapy (a procedure intended to "rescue" a patient after a failed prior therapy) for men who fail to respond to EBRT or interstitial seeds. Ideal candidates are men with a Gleason score < 8. In select cases, cryotherapy may be used as the initial treatment for prostate cancer.

73. What is the success rate of cryotherapy?

In patients who have not responded locally to EBRT, approximately 40% who then undergo salvage cryotherapy have an undetectable PSA level after cryotherapy, and 78% have negative prostate biopsy results. It appears that a drop in the PSA to 0.5 ng/mL after cryotherapy is associated with a good prognosis. In men with postcryotherapy PSA levels > 0.5 ng/mL, there is a higher likelihood that the PSA will increase or that the prostate biopsy result will be positive. When cryotherapy is used as the initial primary therapy, a PSA lowest value of ≤ 0.5 ng/mL is associated with a better prognosis.

The complications of cryotherapy appear to be related to the effects of the freezing on surrounding tissues and can be minimized by careful transrectal ultrasound monitoring and urethral warming during the procedure. Most individuals undergoing cryotherapy are undergoing the treatment as a salvage procedure after failed radiation therapy. The radiation effects on the surrounding tissues leave the tissue with limited reserve for healing and repair, thus increasing the risk of complications.

Common side effects of cryotherapy include perineal pain, transient urinary retention, and hematuria. Urinary retention occurs in roughly 3% of individuals. Stress-related urinary incontinence may occur in up to 20% of individuals, whereas total incontinence occurs

Salvage

A procedure intended to "rescue" a patient after a failed prior therapy, e.g., a salvage radical prostatectomy after failed external-beam therapy.

in only 2%. However, in individuals undergoing salvage cryotherapy after radiation failure, the incidence of urinary incontinence may be as high as 43%. Erectile dysfunction is reported in 40% of individuals undergoing cryotherapy. Rarely, a fistula between the rectum and the urethra may occur.

74. What options are available if primary cryotherapy does not help me?

If the failure occurs locally within the prostate and there is no sign of cancer outside of the prostate, then a radical prostatectomy could technically be performed. The risks of incontinence and impotence associated with radical prostatectomy after cryotherapy are significant. Hormone therapy is also an option in patients with a rising PSA after primary cryotherapy.

75. Are there different types of hormone therapy? Do I need to have my testicles removed?

Hormones

Substances (estrogens and androgens) responsible for secondary sex characteristics (hair growth and voice change in men).

Androgens

Hormones that are necessary for the development and function of the male sexual organs and male sexual characteristics (i.e., hair, voice change).

Hormone therapy is a form of prostate cancer treatment designed to eliminate the male hormones (androgens) from the body. **Hormones** are substances that are responsible for secondary sex characteristics, such as hair growth and voice changes in males. **Androgens** are necessary for the development and function of the male sexual organs and male sexual characteristics (e.g., hair, voice change). The most common androgen is **testosterone**. Androgens are primarily produced by the testicles, under control of various parts of the brain. A small amount of androgens is produced by the adrenal glands, which are small glands located above the kidneys and which produce many important chemicals. Prostate cancer cells may be hormone sensitive, hormone insensitive, or hormone resistant. Cancer cells that are hormone sensitive require androgens for growth. Thus, elimination of the androgens would prevent the growth of such cells and cause them to shrink. Normal prostate cells are also hormone sensitive and also shrink in response to hormone therapy. Prostate cancer cells that are hormone resistant continue to grow despite hormone therapy.

Hormone therapy is not a "curative" therapy, because it does not eliminate the prostate cancer cells; rather, it is "palliative" in that its goal is to slow down the progression, or growth, of the prostate cancer. Hormone therapy for patients with metastatic disease may work effectively for several years; however, over time, the hormone-resistant cells will emerge, and the cancer will grow.

Hormone therapy may be used as a primary, secondary, or neoadjuvant therapy. Hormone therapy is often used as a primary therapy in older men who are not candidates for surgery or radiation therapy and who are not interested in watchful waiting (Question 83). It is also used in men who have metastatic disease at the time that their prostate cancer is detected. Men who experience a rise in their PSA after radical prostatectomy, radiation therapy, or cryotherapy are given hormone therapy to slow down the growth of the recurrent prostate cancer. Lastly, hormone therapy may be given for a period of time before radical prostatectomy or radiation therapy to shrink the prostate gland and make the procedure easier to perform (**neoadjuvant therapy**). It is unclear whether this type of therapy affects the time to disease progression or survival. However, neoadjuvant therapy has a significant impact on the pathology, such that it is very difficult for the pathologist to grade the cancer cells after three months of hormone therapy.

Testosterone

The male hormone or androgen that is produced primarily by the testes and is needed for sexual function and fertility.

Hormone therapy is not a "curative" therapy, because it does not eliminate the prostate cancer cells; rather, it is "palliative" in that its goal is to slow down the progression, or growth, of the prostate cancer.

Neoadjuvant therapy

The use of a treatment, such as chemotherapy, hormone therapy, and radiation therapy, before surgery.

In men with recurrent prostate cancer after EBRT or radical prostatectomy or in those who do not have organ-confined prostate cancer at the time of diagnosis, the time at which hormone therapy should be started is not clear. For this reason, one must weigh the potential benefits and side effects of hormone therapy. Hormone therapy may delay disease progression, but its effect on survival does not appear to be significant. In one study in men with prostate cancer, delaying hormone therapy for one year was associated with an 18% increase risk of death due to prostate cancer; although this was a large study, it is still only one study, and more information is needed.

Many different forms of hormone therapy exist, and they may be subdivided into two groups: surgical and medical therapies. The surgical approach is a bilateral **orchiectomy** (removal of both testicles), whereby the main source of androgen production, the testicles, are removed.

Orchiectomy

Removal of the testicle(s).

Bilateral orchiectomy is performed in men with prostate cancer to remove most of the male hormone (testosterone) production.

Bilateral orchiectomy is performed in men with prostate cancer to remove most of the male hormone (testosterone) production. Typically, this procedure can be performed as a minor surgical procedure under local anesthesia. Depending on the urologist's preference, it can be performed through a single incision in the middle of the scrotum or through two incisions, one on each side of the scrotum. The blood vessels that supply the testis and the sperm duct (the vas deferens) are tied off, and the testes are removed. Some urologists perform a subcapsular orchiectomy, whereby the testicular tissue is removed from within the outer coat (the capsule), and the capsule remains in the scrotum, leaving some fullness to the scrotum. To minimize swelling and bleeding in the scrotum, the scrotum is often wrapped to compress it or a scrotal supporter is used to elevate it. The incision is closed with dissolvable sutures so that the stitches will not need to be removed.

The advantages of bilateral orchiectomy are that it causes a quick drop in the testosterone level (the testosterone level drops to its lowest level by 3 to 12 hours after the procedure [average is 8.6 hours]), it is a one-time procedure, and it is more cost effective than the shots, which require several office visits per year and are more expensive. The disadvantages of orchiectomy are those of any surgical procedure and include bleeding, infection, permanence, and scrotal changes. In men who have undergone bilateral orchiectomy and are bothered by an "empty" scrotum, bilateral testicular prostheses may be placed that are the same size as the adult testes. Most men who undergo bilateral orchiectomy lose their libido and have erectile dysfunction after the testosterone level is lowered. Other long-term side effects of bilateral orchiectomy, related to testosterone depletion, include hot flashes, osteoporosis, fatigue, loss of muscle mass, anemia, and weight gain.

Medical therapy is designed to stop the production of androgens by the testicles. There are three types of medical therapies: **luteinizing hormone-releasing hormone (LHRH) analogues**, **antiandrogens**, and **gonadotropin-releasing hormone (GnRH) antagonists**. These prevent the action of testosterone on the prostate cancer and on normal prostate cells (antiandrogen), or prevent the production of adrenal androgens.

Luteinizing Hormone-Releasing Hormone Analogues

The brain controls testosterone production by the testicles. Leuteinizing hormone-releasing hormone analogues are chemicals produced in the brain that in turn stimulate the production of another chemical produced by the brain, the luteinizing hormone. Luteinizing hormone tells the testicles to produce testosterone. Initially, when a man

Luteinizing hormone-releasing hormone (LHRH) analogues

A class of drugs that prevent testosterone production by the testes.

Antiandrogen

A medication that eliminates or reduces the presence or activity of androgens.

GnRH antagonist

A form of hormone therapy which works at the level of the brain to directly suppress the production of testosterone without initially raising the testosterone level.

takes an LHRH analogue, there is an increased production of LH and of testosterone. This superstimulation in turn tells the brain to stop producing LHRH and, subsequently, the testicles stop producing testosterone. It takes about 5 to 8 days for the LHRH analogues to drop the testosterone levels significantly. The increase in testosterone that may occur initially with LHRH analogues may affect patients with bone metastases, and there may be a worsening of their bone pain called the **flare reaction**. Such men with metastatic disease will be given another medication, an antiandrogen, for two weeks or so before starting the LHRH analogue to block the effects of the testosterone and to prevent the flare phenomenon. An LHRH antagonist is not associated with the flare phenomenon and thus use of an antiandrogen is not needed initially.

Flare reaction

A temporary increase in tumor growth and symptoms that is caused by the initial use of LHRH agonists: It is prevented by the use of an antiandrogen 1 week before LHRH agonist therapy begins.

LHRH analogues are given as shots either monthly, every 3 months, every 4 months, every 6 months, or yearly. There are a variety of LHRH analogues and an LHRH antagonist available, which vary in the frequency of administration and how they are given. The advantage of this form of therapy is that it does not require removal of the testicles; however, it is expensive and requires more frequent visits to the doctor's office. If you miss a shot, your testosterone level increases, and the prostate cancer cells may grow; thus, it is important to get the shots on a regularly scheduled basis. If you are traveling, you can plan ahead and contact doctors in areas where you will be to arrange for the shots.

LHRH analogues have side effects that may affect your quality of life over the short and long term (**Table 8**). Some of the side effects related to these medications, such as hot flashes, erectile dysfunction (see Question 91), anemia, and osteoporosis, can be treated. Erectile dysfunction occurs in about 80% of men taking LHRH analogues and is associated with decreased libido (sexual

Table 8 Antiandrogens and LHRH Analogues

Agent	Route of Administration	Side Effects
LHRH analog	IM, SQ	Impotence, decreased libido, osteoporosis, anemia, hot flashes, weight gain, fatigue, flare phenomenon
LHRH antagonist	IM	Impotence, decreased libido, anemia, hot flashes, weight gain, fatigue
Antiandrogen	Oral	Breast tenderness and enlargement, hot flashes, anemia, abnormal liver function

Abbreviations: SQ, subcutaneously; IM, intramuscularly; Oral, taken orally

desire). Oral therapies for erectile dysfunction, PDE-5 inhibitors, are effective in most of these men if they had normal erectile function before starting hormone therapy. Unfortunately, there is no medication to restore libido.

A recent Gallup survey of American men revealed that most men believe that osteoporosis is "a woman's disease." **Osteoporosis** is loss of bone density, and it leads to weakened bones that break more easily. Yet this disease can affect men, particularly men taking hormone therapy for prostate cancer. It is anticipated that there will be approximately 2,000 osteoporosis-induced fractures in men with advanced prostate cancer.

How can you tell if osteoporosis is occurring? The best way to check the bone mineral density is the dual-energy X-ray absorptiometry (DEXA) scan, the same study used to evaluate for osteoporosis in women. It is **noninvasive** (i.e., it does not require an incision or the insertion of an instrument or substance into the body), precise, and a quick test that involves minimal radiation exposure. The test measures

Osteoporosis

The reduction in the amount of bone mass, leading to fractures after minimal trauma.

Noninvasive

Not requiring any incision or the insertion of an instrument or substance into the body.

the bone mineral density, which is compared with values obtained from normal, young, adult control subjects. The controls have been well established for women but need to be better defined for men. In addition, there appears to be an ethnic variability in bone density, with African-American males usually having higher peak bone mass and a lower risk of osteoporotic fractures than white males. Normally, the bone mineral density is at its highest by age 25, and after age 35 both men and women lose 0.3% to 0.5% of their bone mass per year as part of the normal aging process. Men have a higher peak bone mass than women.

Osteoporosis is loss of bone density, and it leads to weakened bones that break more easily.

Several factors contribute to loss of bone mineral density, but decreased sex hormone production has the most significant impact on bone mineral density. Low testosterone levels affect bone mineral density in men almost the same as low estrogen levels in women. The use of androgen deprivation therapy, whether it be via orchiectomy or LHRH analogue or LHRH antagonist with or without antiandrogen, causes decreased bone mineral density. There is an average loss of 4% per year for the first two years on hormone therapy and 2% per year after year 4, which is similar to the loss in women after removal of the ovaries or natural menopause. This loss of bone mineral density in men taking hormone therapy occurs for at least ten years and probably accounts for the increased incidence of fractures: 5% to 13.5% of men taking hormone therapy have fractures compared to 1% in men with prostate cancer who are not receiving hormone therapy.

Lifestyle modifications that may help decrease the risks of bone complications in men on hormonal therapy include: smoking cessation, decreased alcohol intake, performing weight bearing and arm exercises, and taking supplements of 1200 mg of calcium and 400 to 800 international units of vitamin D daily. Calcium rich diets include dairy products, salmon, spinach and tofu.

When should men on hormone therapy be evaluated for osteoporosis? There are no good guidelines to help determine how frequently DEXA scans should be obtained in men with prostate cancer who are taking hormone therapy. It may be helpful to obtain a baseline DEXA scan before starting hormone therapy and then obtain periodic DEXA scans thereafter. What can be done to prevent or treat osteoporosis? Several studies have shown that an increase in bone mineral density loss occurs in men who have had an orchiectomy compared to men who are receiving LHRH analogues or antagonists. The reason for this is not clear, but this result suggests that other chemicals are produced by the testes that may be important in maintaining bone density. Further studies may help identify these chemicals. Certain factors can put one at increased risk for osteoporosis, including sedentary lifestyle, decreased sun exposure, glucocorticoid therapy, excess caffeine intake, decreased dietary calcium and vitamin D intake or exposure, increased salt intake, aluminum-containing antacid consumption, alcohol abuse, and smoking.

Changes in lifestyle can help prevent osteoporosis. Various medications have been used in women with osteoporosis, but no treatments have been approved by the United States Food and Drug Administration (**FDA**) for men taking hormone therapy. Low-dose estrogen therapy has been shown to be helpful in stabilizing the loss of bone mineral density, but it has the risk of blood clots.

Another group of medications that are more commonly used in women with osteoporosis are the biphosphonates, which prevent bone breakdown. Some have been used to prevent osteoporosis in androgen-deficient men with prostate cancer.

FDA

Food and Drug Administration. Agency responsible for the approval of prescription medications in the United States.

119

Another way of decreasing the risk of osteoporosis is the use of intermittent hormone therapy. With this form of therapy, you are on and off the hormones for set periods of time. The idea of intermittent hormone therapy is that the prostate cancer cells that survive while you are on hormone therapy (hormone insensitive) become hormone sensitive again when they are exposed to androgens. Possible advantages of intermittent androgen suppression include preservation of androgen sensitivity of the tumor, possible prolonged survival, improved quality of life because of recovery of libido and potency and improved sense of well-being, decrease in treatment costs, increased sensitivity of the prostate cancer to chemotherapy, and the fact that it can be used to treat all stages of prostate cancer. Intermittent hormone therapy appears to affect bone mineral density loss at six years.

The long-term effects of intermittent hormone therapy are not well known. The duration that one receives the hormone therapy, the time to restart hormone therapy, how to tell whether the disease is progressing, and who is the ideal patient for intermittent hormone therapy are not well defined. One potential way to give intermittent androgen suppression therapy (androgen blockade) is shown in **Table 9**.

Table 9 Intermittent Androgen Blockage

PSA nadir < 4 ng/mL
　　Continue on therapy for an average of 9 months
　　　　↓
Discontinue medications
　　Watch until PSA increases to mean of 10–20 ng/mL
　　　　↓
Resume androgen blockade
　　Continue cycling until regulation of PSA becomes independent of androgen blockade

LHRH analogues and antagonists often are used alone as primary, secondary, or neoadjuvant therapy. Over time, the PSA level may increase. When the PSA increases, your doctor may check your serum testosterone level to make sure that the LHRH analogue/antagonist is dropping the testosterone level to almost undetectable levels. In some cases with use of the LHRH analogue on an every-3-to 4-month basis, the testosterone suppression may not be adequate, and switching to a more frequent dosing interval, such as an every-28-day formulation, may be more effective. When a man is receiving hormone therapy, the testosterone level should be <20 ng/dL. When the PSA increases despite LHRH analogues/antagonists, the LHRH analogue/antagonist is continued and another medication, an antiandrogen, may be added. This combined therapy is called total androgen blockade and may be effective in treating the prostate cancer for 3 to 6 months. Alternatively, another form of hormonal therapy may be added.

Antiandrogens

Antiandrogens are receptor blockers; they prevent the attachment of the androgens, both those produced by the testicles and those produced by the adrenal glands, to the prostate cancer cells, thus preventing them from acting on these cells. Because these chemicals do not actually affect testosterone production, the testosterone level remains normal or may be slightly elevated if they are used alone. Thus, these medications do not affect libido or erectile function when they are used alone. However, antiandrogens are not commonly used alone; rather, they are used in combination with LHRH analogue/antagonist. As with all medications, these medications have side effects, which are listed in Table 8. When antiandrogens are used in combination with LHRH analogue/antagonist, this is called **total androgen blockade**. Total androgen blockade is used

Antiandrogen

A medication that eliminates or reduces the presence or activity of androgens.

Total androgen blockade

The total blockage of all male hormones (those produced by the testicles and the adrenals) using surgery and/or medications.

Antiandrogens are receptor blockers; they prevent the attachment of the androgens, both those produced by the testicles and those produced by the adrenal glands, to the prostate cancer cells, thus preventing them from acting on these cells.

Hot flashes

The sudden feeling of being warm, may be associated with sweating and flushing of the skin, which occurs with hormone therapy.

for individuals whose PSA increases significantly while they are taking LHRH analogues. LHRH antagonists have been shown to rapidly decrease serum testosterone levels and are not associated with the risk of a flare reaction as seen with the LHRH agonist.

76. Why do hot flashes occur with hormone therapy, and can they be treated?

Hot flashes occur in men receiving hormone therapy for the treatment of high-stage prostate cancer and in patients receiving neoadjuvant hormone therapy (hormone therapy administered before definitive treatment, e.g., radical prostatectomy or interstitial seeds to shrink the prostate cancer).

In a study of men receiving neoadjuvant therapy before radical prostatectomy, **hot flashes** (a sudden feeling of being warm, which may be associated with sweating and flushing of the skin) occurred in 80% of the patients. In about 10%, the hot flashes continued for at least 3 months after they stopped the hormone therapy. Men who received hormone therapy for > 4 months were more likely to have hot flashes that persisted. Approximately three quarters (75%) of the men being treated with hormone therapy for prostate cancer report bothersome hot flashes that begin 1 to 12 months after starting hormone therapy and often persist for years. The hot flashes may vary in intensity and can last from a few seconds to an hour.

The cause of hot flashes and sweating (vasomotor symptoms) associated with hormone therapy (shots or orchiectomy) is not well known. The symptoms are similar to those that women experience while going through menopause, yet they are not typically experienced by men, whose testosterone level slowly declines with aging. The symptoms appear to be related to the sudden large decrease in the testosterone level and the effects that testosterone has on blood vessels. There are no identifiable factors that put one individual at higher risk for hot flashes than another.

There are many ways to treat hot flashes associated with hormone therapy, and different men respond to different treatments. Limiting caffeine intake and avoiding strenuous exercise and very warm temperatures are also helpful in controlling hot flashes.

Hot flashes occur in men receiving hormone therapy for the treatment of high-stage prostate cancer and in patients receiving neoadjuvant hormone therapy

77. What happens when androgen blockade fails and the PSA starts rising again?

If the PSA level increases while you are receiving total androgen blockade, first your doctor will stop the antiandrogen, called "antiandrogen withdrawal." This causes the PSA to decrease in about 20% of cases, and this effect may last for several months to years. The LHRH analogue/antagonist therapy is continued. It is not clear why this antiandrogen withdrawal works. When the PSA rises after antiandrogen withdrawal, you may consider other forms of hormone therapy.

Chemotherapy has an increasing role in the management of men with hormone refractory/resistant prostate cancer (see Question 79). Taxanes have been approved for use for hormone refractory prostate cancer and have been shown to increase survival with manageable side effects. Clinical trials investigating the use of chemotherapeutic drugs for prostate cancer are ongoing. Such trials allow some patients to participate in evaluating the effectiveness and safety of newer forms of chemotherapy (see Question 89). They may or may not be beneficial to you, however, the information that is gained from them allows oncologists to learn more about prostate cancer and effective treatment options.

78. What is hormone-refractory prostate cancer and how does one treat it?

When the PSA continues to increase despite all forms of hormone therapy, your condition is called "hormone refractory," which means that it is resistant to hormone treatment.

In patients with metastatic disease at the time of diagnosis, in those who are too ill for a curative therapy, or in those who develop recurrent prostate cancer after surgery or radiation therapy, hormone therapy is often used. First-line hormone therapy is usually orchiectomy or an LHRH analogue/antagonist. For men in whom the prostate cancer continues to grow while they are receiving first-line hormone therapy, an antiandrogen is added.

Increases in PSA while you are receiving total androgen blockade (orchiectomy or LHRH analogue/antagonist plus antiandrogen) indicate the presence of hormone-insensitive prostate cancer cells. If this occurs, the antiandrogen is withdrawn, and the LHRH analogue/antagonist is continued. When the PSA continues to increase despite this change, another form of hormone therapy may be used. When the PSA continues to increase despite all forms of hormone therapy, your condition is called "hormone refractory," which means that it is resistant to hormone treatment. In this situation, the option is chemotherapy, either a current FDA-approved regimen or a clinical trial that evaluates newer medications or newer doses or combinations of therapies (see Question 89).

Hormone refractory

Prostate cancer that is resistant to hormone therapy.

79. Is chemotherapy used for prostate cancer?

Chemotherapy is the use of powerful drugs either to kill cancer cells or interfere with their growth. Many different types of chemotherapeutic agents work at different times in the growth cycle of the cell, and combinations of agents often are used to maximize the effects on the cancer cells. Several different drugs have been shown to improve symptoms and decrease the PSA level or the amount of cancer, though no drug has been shown to kill all of the prostate cancer cells present. Ongoing clinical trials continue to look at new chemotherapy drugs, combinations of drugs, or different doses in hopes of finding more effective and less toxic options.

A variety of chemotherapies have been tried in individuals when hormone therapy fails. Some doctors question whether patients would respond better to chemotherapy if used earlier in the disease when the cells are hormone responsive.

Several ongoing studies sponsored by the National Cancer Institute and the National Institutes of Health are evaluating the use of various chemotherapy regimens for hormone-refractory prostate cancer. To find out about these studies and their eligibility criteria, ask your urologist or oncologist to help you identify which of these agents may be best for you or call the nearest cancer center.

80. When should one start chemotherapy?

If prostate cancer reappears despite surgery, or no longer responds to hormonal therapy, a medical oncologist should join the treatment team because he or she may use chemotherapy. He or she helps you plan chemotherapy and takes charge of chemotherapy treatment. Regardless of whether you are or are not experiencing pain or discomfort from your cancer, you should consult your medical oncologist once hormone therapy is no longer effective. The risks and benefits of chemotherapy and the expected results should be discussed with your doctor so that you may decide if and when you are ready to begin chemotherapy.

81. What is vaccine therapy for prostate cancer?

Vaccine therapy involves the injection of a chemical, an antigen, into an individual. The antigen stimulates the individual's body to produce cells that fight off the antigen and, in doing so, kill the cancer cells. Several different vaccine therapies are being investigated, but none are currently available.

82. What is gene therapy for prostate cancer?

Prostate cells become malignant because of gene changes in the cells. The goal of gene therapy is to place genes into the cancer cells that would cause the cancer cells to return to their normal state or would cause the cancer cells to die. Various centers throughout the United States are running clinical trials using gene therapy: the Johns Hopkins University School of Medicine, UCLA

Medical Center, Duke University Medical Center, University of Michigan School of Medicine, Dana Farber Cancer Institute, Baylor College of Medicine, Mt. Sinai School of Medicine, Vanderbilt University Medical Center, and MD Anderson Cancer Center.

83. What is watchful waiting?

Watchful waiting is the decision not to treat the prostate cancer at the time of diagnosis and is not aimed at curing one of prostate cancer, but rather to institute palliative treatment for local or metastatic disease progression if it occurs. Rather than treat the cancer, the physician monitors the PSA value at various intervals to assess whether it is increasing and at what rate (the **PSA velocity**). Ideally, the patient and the physician identify a point at which therapy would be instituted (for example, a PSA value of a certain number or the presence of bone pain), and the patient is monitored without therapy until he changes his mind or that point is reached. Watchful waiting differs from active surveillance in that with active surveillance one is followed more closely and the intent is to intervene while the prostate cancer may still be treated definitively.

Watchful waiting is ideally suited for patients with potentially life-threatening medical conditions and older patients with low Gleason scores. In these individuals, it is less likely that prostate cancer will be the cause of their death. Younger (< 72 years) men, healthy men, and those with a higher Gleason score are more likely to live long enough to have symptoms and disease progression in their lifetime and are better suited to more definitive treatment if the cancer is identified early at a low stage.

Watchful waiting
Active observation and regular monitoring of a patient without actual treatment.

PSA velocity
The rate of change of the PSA over a period of time (change in PSA ÷ change in time).

Watchful waiting is ideally suited for patients with potentially life-threatening medical conditions and older patients with low Gleason scores.

Two large ongoing clinical trials are designed to compare watchful waiting with radical prostatectomy in men with clinically localized prostate cancer. The trial in the United States is the U.S. Prostate Cancer Intervention Versus Observation Trial (PIVOT). There is also a study comparing watchful waiting with radiation therapy for clinically localized prostate cancer (RIVOT). If you are interested in participating in this study, the radiation oncology department in your hospital should be able to direct you to a participating center.

Pros of Watchful Waiting

Morbidity

Unhealthy results and complications resulting from treatment

1. **Morbidity**, meaning unhealthy results and complications of active treatment (e.g., incontinence, erectile dysfunction), is significant, especially in younger men.

2. Risk of cancer progression with low-grade, low-stage tumor is low (10–25%) within ten years.

3. Rarely does low-grade, low-stage disease advance within five years.

Cons of Watchful Waiting

1. In men with nonmetastatic disease who survive more than 10 years, 63% die of prostate cancer.

2. In younger patients with initially confined disease who undergo watchful waiting, there is a higher risk of developing incurable disease and dying from it.

84. What is potency-sparing therapy for prostate cancer?

Unfortunately, most treatments of prostate cancer carry the risk of permanent erectile dysfunction, which may have a significant impact on one's quality of life. Many men have chosen radiation therapy (either interstitial seeds or EBRT) because the risk of erectile dysfunction may be less and the onset is slower than with surgery. Early use of hormone therapy in men who are at high risk for recurrence after definitive therapies and in men who are not candidates for surgery or radiation therapy also has long-term effects on erectile function. Currently, antiandrogens are not FDA approved for use as a single therapy for prostate cancer. 5-alpha-reductase inhibitors prevent conversion of testosterone to a more active chemical, dihydrotestosterone. They have been shown to shrink benign prostate tissue and lower PSA. Their effect on prostate cancer is being evaluated.

The use of potency-sparing therapies is still considered investigational at this time, and if you are interested in such a therapy, it would be best to contact an academic (teaching) hospital in your area to see if they have any ongoing clinical trials of potency-sparing therapies. Another way to preserve erectile dysfunction and libido, at least partially, is to use intermittent hormone therapy (see Question 75). With intermittent hormone therapy, erectile function is usually restored during the times that you are not taking the hormone therapy.

85. What alternative therapies are available for prostate cancer?

Alternative medicine, or treatment that is different from accepted therapies, is commonly used in the United States, where more visits are made to alternative health providers than to primary care providers.

Alternative treatment

The treatment is used instead of accepted treatments.

The most commonly used alternative therapies are acupuncture, biofeedback, chiropractic, energy healing, herbal medicine, homeopathy, hypnosis, imagery, massage, relaxation techniques, and vitamins and minerals.

Acupuncture

A Chinese therapy involving the use of thin needles inserted into specific locations in the skin.

Acupuncture is based on the belief that pathways of energy flow through the body that are essential for health and that changes in this flow can cause disease or illness. An acupuncturist uses needles to redirect or correct inadequate energy flow. On a more scientific basis, it appears that placement of the needle in a certain location causes the release of chemicals from nerves that may alter one's perception of pain or cause the release of other chemicals that may affect perception of pain and may also improve healing. The National Institutes of Health have approved the use of acupuncture for relief of postoperative pain and treatment of nausea associated with chemotherapy. Its use in advanced-stage prostate cancer has possible advantages and disadvantages:

Advantages

- It may help relieve cancer-related pain.
- It may help relieve chemotherapy-induced nausea.
- It may affect the **immune response** (the response of organs, tissues, blood cells, and substances that fight off infections, cancers, or foreign substances) to cancer.

Immune response

The response of organs, tissues, blood cells, and substances that fight off infections, cancers, or foreign substances.

- It tends to promote more self-control and involvement by the patient in his treatment.
- It may be covered by some managed care and insurance companies.
- Side effects are minimal if the acupuncturist is well-trained.

Disadvantages

- Limited studies are available comparing a **placebo** (a fake medication or treatment that has no effect on the body) with acupuncture.
- No specific studies are available regarding the use of acupuncture in advanced prostate cancer.
- The patient needs to assess whether the acupuncturist is well-trained because there are no specific training requirements in most states.
- If the acupuncturist is inexperienced, there is a risk of infection and injury.

If you are interested in acupuncture as a therapy for nausea, consult with your doctor—he or she might have a list of approved practitioners in your area. If not, the American Academy of Medical Acupuncture keeps a list of accredited practitioners nationwide, know the laws governing the practice for your state, and has information regarding how acupuncture should be used. Contact information for the AAMA can be found in the Appendix.

Dietary Therapies

Lycopene is a carotenoid that is found in tomatoes and is a strong antioxidant. It has been shown to decrease the risk of prostate cancer. Several small studies have suggested a role for lycopene supplementation in men with

The most commonly used alternative therapies are acupuncture, biofeedback, chiropractic, energy healing, herbal medicine, homeopathy, hypnosis, imagery, massage, relaxation techniques, and vitamins and minerals.

Placebo

A fake medication ("candy pill") or treatment that has no effect on the body that is often used in experimental studies to determine if the experimental medication/treatment has an effect.

131

prostate cancer; however, further studies are needed to determine whether or not it is truly effective.

Soy products are high in isoflavones, which have been shown to prevent cancer cell growth. The effects of soy supplementation in both prostate cancer prevention and in men with prostate cancer are being studied.

Herbal Remedies

It is important to note that herbal remedies sometimes have interactions with other medications or treatments, so you should never begin taking them without first consulting with your doctor. Herbal preparations are not monitored for purity by the FDA, so be cautious about what you buy; check the information on the label, and investigate the brands' reputations before you choose one.

86. When can I consider myself cured of prostate cancer?

Prostate cancer, like all cancers, does not "play by the rules." It does not reach out to areas outside of the prostate in a straight line such that if no cancer is present at the edge of the prostate then no cancer exists at all outside of the prostate. Cancer cells may remain in the pelvis, get into the bloodstream, or be present in the bones and not grow quickly enough for them to be noticed for several years. In the strictest sense, a cancer is considered to be "cured" when there is no evidence of any cancer ten years after treatment. This seems like an awfully long time, and certainly you do not need to hold your breath and put your life on hold during this time; the PSA testing along the way will help assure you that all is going well. PSA testing is the most sensitive way of detecting a recurrence of the prostate cancer and detects it sooner than bone scans or other types of X-ray studies. With radical prostatectomy, the PSA decreases to an undetectable level in most people because the producer of PSA, the prostate, has been removed. Rarely, small glands in the urethra may produce very small amounts of PSA, which may account for a PSA level that is slightly above undetectable but does not increase over time. With radiation therapy, both interstitial seeds and EBRT, the prostate is not removed, and thus the PSA does not decrease to an undetectable range. The PSA will drop, however, reflecting the death of the cancer cells and the loss of PSA production. It should drop to ≤ 0.5 ng/dL and remain at that level thereafter. Biopsy of the prostate is not routinely used to confirm that treatment has been effective after interstitial seed therapy or EBRT, because the changes that occur in the cells after radiation therapy make interpretation of the biopsy very difficult. The PSA is more helpful in this situation.

PART SIX

Complications of Treatment

Are there any predictors of recurrence of prostate cancer after "curative" therapy?

What happens if the PSA is rising after radiation therapy or radical prostatectomy?

My doctor has recommended that I be involved in a clinical trial. What is a clinical trial?

More . . .

87. Are there any predictors of recurrence of prostate cancer after "curative" therapy?

If one undergoes a radical prostatectomy, the surgical margins, the Gleason score, and the preoperative and postoperative PSA are good predictors of the likelihood of recurrence. The higher the preoperative prostate biopsy Gleason score (7 and higher) and PSA (>20 ng/mL), the higher the likelihood of prostate cancer progression after surgery. For patients with prostate cancer that is pathologically confined to the prostate, the likelihood of being prostate cancer free as determined by PSA level is >90%. A Gleason score of the prostate specimen of 8 or higher is associated with an increased risk of prostate cancer progression. A researcher at Stanford University looked at the percent of high-grade cancer in the prostate specimen and found that the higher the percent of Gleason grade 4 or 5 in the tumor, the higher the risk of a rising postoperative PSA. The Gleason score and the initial PSA are also predictors of success of EBRT and interstitial seed therapy. Several clinical factors are useful in predicting the site of recurrence after radical prostatectomy (**Table 10**).

88. What happens if the PSA is rising after radiation therapy or radical prostatectomy?

PSA progression

Increase in PSA after treatment of prostate cancer.

Biochemical progression

Recurrence of prostate cancer as defined by an elevation in PSA.

When the PSA rises after definitive therapy, such as EBRT, interstitial seed therapy, and radical prostatectomy, it is called **PSA progression**. In the absence of any identifiable cancer, it is called **biochemical progression**, because the only indicator of progression of the cancer is the PSA level. When the PSA is increasing

Table 10 Clinical Factors Useful in Predicting the Anatomic Site of Recurrence After Radical Prostatectomy

Clinical Factor	Site of Recurrence	
	Local	**Distant**
Time of PSA recurrence	> 2 years	< 2 years
PSA doubling time (Trap)	> 12 months	< 6 months
PSA velocity (Partin)	≤ 0.75 ng/mL/year	> 0.75 ng/mL/year
Pathologic stage	Capsular penetration or positive surgical margins	Seminal vesicle or lymph node involvement
Pathologic grade	Gleason score < 7	Gleason score ≥ 7

Reprinted with permission from *Urol Clinics N Am* 1998; 25:593.

after definitive therapy, your physician may want to re-stage you to determine where the cancer is. It is helpful in the decision making to determine whether the prostate cancer is confined to the prostate (in men who have had interstitial seed therapy or EBRT), the area where the prostate was (in post–radical prostatectomy patients), or the pelvis, or whether it has spread outside of the prostatic area, for example, to the bones or lymph nodes higher up in your abdomen. Methods used in this staging process may be a bone scan (see Question 43), a ProstaScint scan (see Question 45), and/or a CT scan of the abdomen and pelvis. In certain cases, the doctor may recommend a biopsy of the prostate, of the bladder neck area, or of other areas that may be likely to have cancer.

When the PSA rises after radical prostatectomy, the relevant question is whether there is **local recurrence** of the prostate cancer (return of the cancer to the area where it was first identified) or distant disease to the area where it was first identified (metastatic disease). Overall, about 30% of men with detectable PSA levels after

Local recurrence

The return of cancer to the area where it was first identified.

radical prostatectomy have local recurrences, whereas about 70% are anticipated to have distant disease alone or distant disease combined with local disease. The timing of the PSA recurrence, the rate of the rise in PSA, and the pathological stage and grade of the prostate cancer are helpful in predicting the site of the recurrence (Table 10). Currently, a PSA ≥ 0.4 ng/mL after a radical prostatectomy is considered a likely indication of prostate cancer recurrence. Several options are available, including watchful waiting, EBRT, and hormone therapy.

Watchful Waiting

In one study, watchful waiting was used in men with a rising PSA after radical prostatectomy, and they were monitored until they had evidence of metastases. About 8 years after the radical prostatectomy, these men developed metastases, and an additional 5 years later, they died from their prostate cancer. In general, when watchful waiting is used for PSA progression after radical prostatectomy, the PSA is checked on an every 3- to 6-month basis to determine how quickly the PSA is rising (PSA velocity). If the **doubling time**, the time that it takes for the PSA level to double, is long (a year or longer), then the tumor is slow growing. If the doubling time is short (every three months), then the tumor is fast growing, and the patient would probably benefit from early treatment as opposed to continuing with watchful waiting.

Doubling time

The amount of time that it takes for the cancer to double in size.

EBRT

EBRT is used in men with rising PSA levels after radical prostatectomy who are believed to have a local recurrence in the pelvis. It is not helpful if the cancer is highly likely to be outside of the pelvis. Some data suggest that EBRT is most helpful in men in whom the PSA is

< 1.5 to 2.0 ng/mL and that at least 6400 cGY of radiation should be used. Men with low- or moderate-grade cancers (Gleason sum < 7), with tumor in the prostate capsule or at the surgical margin in whom the PSA rises more than two years after the radical prostatectomy, or with a PSA doubling time of > 12 months, seem likely to have a local recurrence and are good candidates for salvage EBRT.

Hormone Therapy

Hormone therapy tends to be used more commonly for men with recurrent cancer in whom the recurrence is believed to be outside of the pelvic area. Although hormone therapy may delay the progression of the prostate cancer, its impact on survival in this situation is not well known. Men with high-grade tumors (Gleason sum > 7) or with cancer in the seminal vesicles or lymph nodes at the time of radical prostatectomy and in whom the PSA rises within two years after prostatectomy most likely have distant disease and are candidates for hormone therapy or watchful waiting.

Treatment of Rising PSA after EBRT

If the PSA rises after EBRT, the options include salvage prostatectomy, salvage cryotherapy, hormone therapy, and watchful waiting. The decision regarding the most appropriate therapy is based on the likelihood of the cancer being confined to the prostate.

Salvage Prostatectomy after EBRT

The ideal patient for a salvage radical prostatectomy after EBRT is one who is believed to have had prostate-confined disease initially at the time of EBRT and who is still believed to have organ-confined disease. Individuals in this group include those who have a Gleason score ≤ 6, a low pretreatment PSA level (< 10 ng/mL), and low clinical stage tumor (T1c or T2a). At the time of the salvage prostatectomy, they should still have a favorable Gleason score, a low clinical stage, and, ideally, a PSA that is < 4 ng/mL. Salvage prostatectomy is a challenging procedure, and if you are considering this option, you should seek out a urologist who has experience with it because there is an increased risk of urinary incontinence, erectile dysfunction, and rectal injury with this procedure. Rarely, because of extensive scarring, it is necessary to remove the bladder in addition to the prostate, and a urinary diversion would be necessary. A urinary diversion is a procedure that allows urine to be diverted to a segment of bowel that can be made into a storage unit similar to a bladder or allows urine to pass out of an opening in the belly wall into a bag, similar to a colostomy.

Salvage Cryotherapy

One of the main uses of cryotherapy is in patients with a rising PSA after EBRT. In patients who have not responded locally to EBRT, approximately 40% of the patients who then undergo salvage cryotherapy will have an undetectable PSA level after cryotherapy, and 78% will have negative prostate biopsy results. It appears that a drop in the PSA to ≤ 0.5 ng/mL after cryotherapy is associated with a good prognosis. In men with postcryotherapy PSA levels > 0.5 ng/mL, there is a higher likelihood that the PSA will increase or that the prostate biopsy result will be positive (see Questions 71 through 73).

Hormone Therapy and Watchful Waiting

Use of these two options in patients with a rising PSA after EBRT is similar to their use in those with a rising PSA after radical prostatectomy.

Treatment of Rising PSA after Interstitial Seed Therapy

Treatment options for a rising PSA after interstitial seed therapy include salvage prostatectomy, EBRT, watchful waiting, and hormone therapy. It is important to remember that after interstitial seed therapy, there may be a benign rise in the PSA level, and this should not be misconstrued as being indicative of recurrent prostate cancer. In both interstitial seed and radiation therapy, for a rising PSA to be indicative of recurrent/ persistent prostate cancer, it must rise sequentially on three occasions at least two weeks apart. The treatment options are dependent on the likelihood of the disease being confined to the prostate. Salvage prostatectomy for interstitial seed failure carries the same risks as with EBRT failures. The ability to use EBRT depends on the amount of radiation that was delivered at the time of the interstitial seeds and the likelihood of the disease being confined to the prostate.

89. My doctor has recommended that I be involved in a clinical trial. What is a clinical trial?

A **clinical trial** is a carefully planned experiment that is designed to evaluate the use of treatment or a medication for an unproven use. Through the use of clinical trials, investigators assess newer ideas in the treatment of various diseases. There are three different types of clinical trials, each with a particular goal. Typically, when a new medication or therapy is being introduced, its evaluation proceeds in an orderly process through each of these trials.

Clinical trials

A carefully planned experiment to evaluate a treatment or medication (often a new drug) for an unproven use.

141

Phase I trials are preliminary short-duration studies that involve only a few patients. These studies are used to see whether the medication or therapy has any effect or any serious side effects. *Phase II* trials involve a larger number of patients and are designed to determine the most active dose of the therapy as well as its side effects. *Phase III* trials involve large numbers of patients and compare the new therapy with the current standard or the best available therapy.

90. What happens if I develop bone pain?

When prostate cancer metastasizes, it tends to travel to the pelvic lymph nodes first and then to the bones. Bone metastases may be silent, meaning that they do not cause any pain, or they may be symptomatic, causing pain or leading to a fracture. Bone metastases are typically identified on a bone scan and can also be seen on a plain X-ray.

There are many ways to treat bone pain. Your doctor will likely try the simplest treatments and those associated with the least side effects first, and then progress as needed. Nonsteroidal anti-inflammatories such as ibuprofen are typically used as a first-line treatment. If the pain is not controlled with these, then narcotics are added. For patients with a localized bone metastasis that is causing persistent discomfort, localized EBRT may be used (EBRT is not useful for men with multiple bone metastases). EBRT provides pain relief in 80% to 90% of patients, and the relief may last for up to one year in slightly more than half of these men. Usually, the total radiation dose is given over 5 to 15 quick treatment sessions.

The side effects of localized EBRT vary with the area that is being irradiated. Treatment of metastases to the skull may cause hair loss and flaking and redness of the scalp. Treatment of cervical spine (neck bone) metastases may cause discomfort with swallowing and hoarseness. If the mid-spine is treated, nausea and vomiting may result. Treatment of pelvic bone metastases may cause diarrhea. Treatment side effects often resolve with time.

When multiple painful bone metastases are present, **hemibody radiation** may be used. Because this therapy affects a larger area of the body, there are more side effects, including lowering of the blood pressure (hypotension), nausea, vomiting, diarrhea, lung irritation, hair loss, and lowering of the blood count. Hemibody radiation is also given over several treatment sessions. It can lead to pain control that lasts up to one year in as many as 70% of individuals.

Hemibody
Half of the body.

Another form of therapy for multiple painful bone metastasis is radioisotope therapy. With this form of therapy, a radioisotope, a chemical that has a radioactive component to it, is injected into a vein. The chemicals used preferentially go to bone that is affected by cancer. These chemicals are picked up by the bone and "radiate" the area.

Biphosphonates are chemicals that interfere with bone breakdown and are typically used for treatment of osteoporosis. Most prostate cancer bone metastases are not "lytic" metastases (i.e., they do not cause bone breakdown), but some bone breakdown does appear to occur; biphosphonates lead to improvement in bone symptoms in men with prostate cancer. Their use in bone pain remains investigational.

Biphosphonate

A type of medication that is used to treat osteoporosis and the bone pain caused by some types of cancer.

91. What is erectile dysfunction (ED), and what happens if I have ED after treatment for my prostate cancer?

Cliff's comment:

When I was told that there were two major long-term risks of surgery, loss of control of urine and erectile dysfunction, I can remember thinking that I can live with impotence but please God, don't let me be incontinent of urine. Well, I underwent a unilateral nerve-sparing prostatectomy, and although I do not get spontaneous erections on my own, I am happy that the "pill" works. "Does it give you the same strength and endurance that you had years ago?" you may ask. I ask, "Does anything you do in your 60s have the same strength and endurance it had years ago?" I am very happy with the oral therapy, and it has remedied my erectile troubles.

Erectile dysfunction is the consistent inability to achieve adequate penile rigidity for penetration or adequate duration of rigidity for completion of sexual performance. Approximately 50% of men 40 to 70 years of age experience erectile dysfunction. To achieve an adequate erection, you must have properly functioning nerves, arteries, and veins. When you are stimulated or aroused, your brain releases chemicals that tell the nerves in the pelvis to release chemicals that in turn tell the arteries in the penis to open and increase blood flow into the penis. At the same time that blood is moving into the penis, the veins in the penis collapse so that the blood remains in the penis, making it rigid and allowing the rigidity to last. Anything that can affect the brain, nerves, arteries, or veins can cause trouble with erections. More common causes of erectile dysfunction include strokes; spinal cord injury; Parkinson's disease; high cholesterol levels; heart disease; poor circulation in the legs; high blood pressure and medications used to treat high blood pressure; depression and medications used to treat depression; diabetes; surgery, such as radical prostatectomy and colorectal cancer surgeries; pelvic radiation; and hormone therapy for prostate cancer.

When seeking treatment for prostate cancer, many men are very concerned about the effects of the treatment on erectile function. Basically, all of the treatment options carry a risk of erectile dysfunction; however, they differ in how soon after treatment the erectile dysfunction occurs and how likely it is to occur. If you are already having trouble with erections, none of the treatments for prostate cancer will improve your erections. The incidence of erectile dysfunction associated with radical prostatectomy varies with patient age, erectile function before surgery, nerve-sparing status, and the surgeon's technical ability to perform a nerve-sparing radical prostatectomy. The incidence of erectile dysfunction after a nerve-sparing radical prostatectomy varies from 16% to 82%. When it occurs with radical prostatectomy, erectile dysfunction is immediate and is related to damage of the pelvic nerves, which travel along the outside edge of the prostate. Men who have undergone nerve-sparing radical prostatectomies who are impotent after surgery may experience return of their erectile function over the following 12 months.

The incidence of erectile dysfunction after EBRT ranges from 32% to 67% and is caused by radiation-related damage to the arteries. Unlike with surgery, the erectile dysfunction occurs a year or more after the radiation. The incidence of erectile dysfunction is 15% to 31% in the first year after EBRT and 40% to 62% at five years after EBRT.

The incidence of erectile dysfunction after interstitial seed therapy with or without medium-dose EBRT ranges from 6% to 50%. Similar to EBRT, the erectile dysfunction tends to occur later than with radical prostatectomy.

Hormone therapy with the LHRH analogues or orchiectomy also causes erectile dysfunction, as well as loss of interest in sex (libido) in most men. This loss of libido is related to the loss of testosterone, but why the loss of testosterone causes troubles with erections is not well known.

Penile prosthesis

A device that is surgically placed into the penis which allows an impotent individual to have an erection.

Various therapies are available for the treatment of erectile dysfunction, including oral, intraurethral, and injection therapies; the vacuum device; and the **penile prosthesis**, which is a device that is surgically placed into the penis that allows an impotent individual to have an erection. (**Table 11**). Oral therapies, PDE-5 inhibitors alone or in combination with other medications, that increase blood flow work in a similar fashion to increase blood flow to the penis during sexual stimulation. Injection therapies do not require sexual stimulation to be effective. Nerve grafting, whereby a nerve is removed from another area of the body and sewn into the site where the pelvic nerve was removed, is being evaluated.

In the treatment of post–radical prostatectomy erectile dysfunction, the effectiveness of oral PDE-5 therapies varies with nerve-sparing status:

Bilateral nerve sparing: 71% success rate

Unilateral nerve sparing: 50% success rate

Non–nerve sparing: 15% success rate

In men with EBRT-associated erectile dysfunction, oral PDE-5 inhibitors works in about 71%. Lastly, in men who have erectile dysfunction associated with interstitial seed therapy, oral PDE-5 inhibitors have a success rate of approximately 80%. PDE-5 inhibitors require sexual stimulation/foreplay and functioning pelvic nerves in order to be effective. It prevents the breakdown of chemicals released by the pelvic nerves; thus, there is more chemical around to tell the arteries in the penis to open up. To be effective, it must be taken about ½ penile prosthesis to 1 ½ hours before sexual stimulation and intercourse.

PDE-5 inhibitors are not for everyone, and you should consult with your doctor before taking any of these medications. Men with unstable angina who use nitroglycerin on a daily or frequent basis should not take any of these medications, nor should men with poorly functioning hearts (congestive heart failure) or men who have high blood pressure that requires several medications to control (Table 11).

Another drug that is used to treat erectile dysfunction is intraurethral PGE-1, a small pellet that comes preloaded in an applicator (**Figure 16**). To use intraurethral PGE-1, you should void first to lubricate the urethra with urine before you insert the applicator. Other lubricants, such as K-Y Jelly® and Vaseline®, cannot be used be used for this purpose. The applicator is placed into the tip of the penis, and the small button at the other end is pressed (**Figure 17**), thus releasing a small suppository. Gentle rubbing of the penis dissolves the suppository in the urethra, and the medication is absorbed. The most common side effect of intraurethral PGE-1 is urethral/penile burning or pain, and men who have undergone a radical prostatectomy seem to have an increased incidence of this side

Table 11 Treatment Options for Erectile Dysfunction

Rx	Administration	Success Rate	Contraindications	Side Effects	Mechanisms of Action
Oral PDE-5 Inhibitors	Oral	48–81%	Retinitis pigmentosa, nitrate use. When using concomitant alpha-blockers, must be stable on alpha-blocker therapy and start with lowest dose of PDE-5 inhibitor. Follow Princeton guidelines regarding use in CV patients.	HA, facial flushing, dyspepsia. NAION (nonarteritic anterior ischemic optic neuropathy) has been reported in individuals taking PDE 5 inhibitors. Risk factors for NAION are similar to those for ED, such as age > 50 yr, HT, increased cholesterol, and DM. Another risk factor is a small cup-to-disk ratio. Pts should be advised to seek medical attention in the event of a sudden loss of vision in one or both eyes. Hearing loss has also been reported in patients taking PDE5 inhibitors. As with NAION a causal relationship has not been established.	Phosphodiesterase type V inhibitor leads to increased cGMP, which stimulates cavernous small muscle relaxation
Intraurethral prostaglandin E1	Small suppository placed into distal urethra via small applicator	30–66% success rate (Nejm 1997; 336:1)	Hypersensitivity to PGE1, pregnant partner, predisposition to priapism (leukemia, multiple myeloma, sickle cell)	Pain (penile, urethral, testicular, perineal) in 33%, lowers blood pressure in 3%, priapism, vaginal irritation in 10%	Absorbed through urethral mucosa and stimulates arterial dilation and flow

Rx	Administration	Success Rate	Contraindications	Side Effects	Mechanisms of Action
Intracavernous injection therapy with prostaglandin E1	Direct injection into lateral aspect of corpora cavernosa, alternating sides with each injection	Average success rate 73% (Int J Impot Res 1994;6:149; J Urol 1988; 140:66)	Known hypersensitivity to prostaglandin E1. Pts at risk for priapism. Pts at increased risk: those on anticoagulants and with Peyronie's dz	Prolonged erections in 1.1–1.3%, corporal fibrosis in 2.7%, painful erection in 15–30%, hematoma, ecchymosis in 1.5%	Prostaglandin E1 stimulates cavernous small muscle relaxation, causes modulation of adenyl cyclase, increase in cAMP and subsequent free Ca^{2+} conc
Vacuum constriction device	Plastic cylinder with hand- or battery-operated pump and constricting bands	68–83% satisfaction rate	Painful ejaculation: 3–16%, inability to ejaculate: 12–30%, petechiae of penis: 25–39%, numbness during erection: 5% (J Urol 1993;149:290; Spahn M, Manning M, Juenemann KP. Textbook of Erectile Dysfunction) Carson C, Kirby R, Goldstein I. Oxford: Isis Medical Media 1999. Intracavernosal therapy.	Use with caution in pts taking aspirin or anticoagulants	Vacuum device creates negative pressure that pulls blood into corpora cavernosa; constriction band prolongs erection by decreasing corporal venous drainage

(continues)

Table 11 Treatment Options for Erectile Dysfunction (Continued)

Rx	Administration	Success Rate	Contraindications	Side Effects	Mechanisms of Action
Penile prosthesis	Surgically placed, models range from semirigid to inflatable	> 90% satisfaction with inflatable prostheses (J Urol 1993; 150:1814; 1992;147:62)	Decreases penile length by 1 cm. Infection < 10%, diabetics at increased risk. Mechanical malfunction < 5% (Urol Clin North Am 1995;22:847). Erosion: increased risk in diabetics and spinal cord injury pts	Requires counseling, preoperative	Cylinders placed in corpora cavernosa provide penile rigidity; once placed, there is corporal fibrosis; if removed, remaining options less likely to work

Adapted from: Ellsworth P, Caldamone, A. *The Little Black Book of Urology*, 2nd ed. Sudbury, MA; Jones and Bartlett Publishers; 2007:181–189.

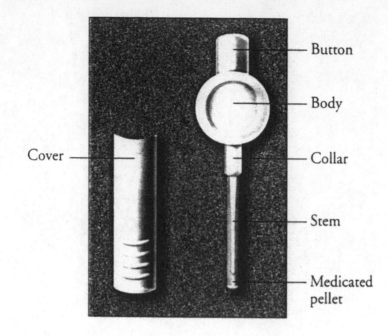

Button

Body

Cover

Collar

Stem

Medicated pellet

Figure 16 Intraurethral prostaglandin E1.
Reprinted with permission from VIVUS, Inc.

effect. Intraurethral PGE-1 works in 20% to 40% of men with post–radical prostatectomy erectile dysfunction.

The vacuum device is composed of several parts: a plastic tube that has a constricting band loaded on it and a pump, either hand-held or battery operated (**Figure 18**) The plastic tube with the preloaded constricting band is placed over the lubricated penis. The pump is then activated, causing a suction that pulls blood into the penis. When the penis is rigid, the constricting band is pulled off of the tube so that it is positioned around the base of the penis; this band serves to hold the blood in the penis. When intercourse is completed, the band is removed, and the blood drains out of the penis. The band should be removed within 30 minutes after placement to

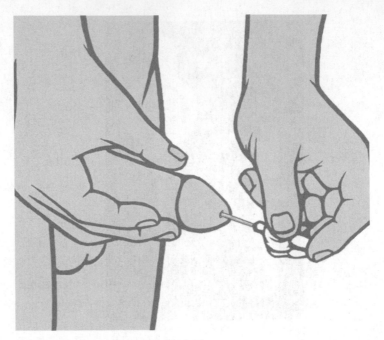

Figure 17 Intraurethral PGE-1 insertion.
© 2002 The StayWell Company. Reprinted with permission.

prevent damage to the penis. The band may affect the ability to ejaculate, but won't affect the orgasm (ability to climax). In men who have had a radical prostatectomy, there will be no fluid (ejaculate), at the time of orgasm. Men who have had EBRT or interstitial seed therapy still have an ejaculate, but the volume may be diminished.

Injection therapy sounds much more painful than it actually is. It involves using a very tiny needle and injecting a small amount of a fluid into the side of the penis (**Figure 19**). The most commonly used form of injection therapy is prostaglandin E1.

Approximately 30% of men experience discomfort with the prostaglandin E1; these individuals can try a combination therapy, such as a combination of phentolamine,

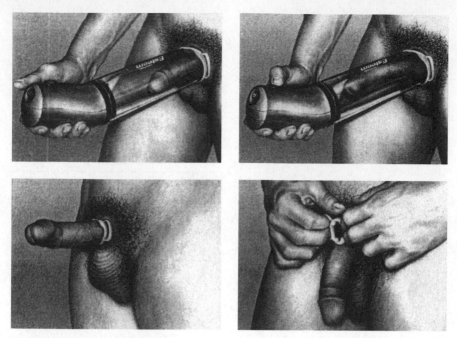

Figure 18 The vacuum device.
Reprinted with permission from Timm Medical Technologies, Inc.

papaverine, and prostaglandin, which contains less prostaglandin. The combination associated with less pain but tends to cause more scarring in the penis than prostaglandin E1 alone. These chemicals tell the blood vessels to open up and increase blood flow into the penis. They work within 10 to 20 minutes after the injection and ideally produce an erection that lasts an hour or so.

Injection therapy works in more than 85% of men with post–radical prostatectomy erectile dysfunction. It may be used in men who have undergone nerve-sparing radical prostatectomies while they await the return of nerve function. In fact, some small studies suggest that early use of injection therapy after radical prostatectomy may quicken the recovery of nerve function. Injection therapy is also very successful in post–EBRT and post–seed placement erectile dysfunction. There is a small

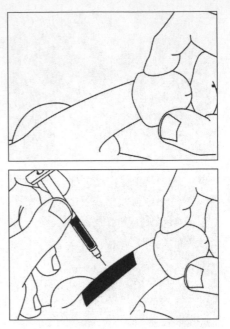

Figure 19
Injection therapy: proper
location of injection.
Reprinted with permission from
Pharmacia-UpJohn.

Priapism

An erection that
lasts longer than 4 to
6 hours.

risk (2%) that the erection produced may last longer than 4 to 6 hours; this condition is called **priapism**. If you experience an erection that lasts longer than 3 to 4 hours, you should call the urologist on call because this condition needs to be treated immediately; otherwise, pain or damage to the penis could result, and the condition becomes more difficult to treat. If you seek help early, then all the doctor may have to do is inject another chemical into the penis to tell the blood vessels to shut down. When performing injection therapy, you should alternate sides of the penis and not perform the injections any more frequently than every 48 to 72 hours to prevent scar tissue from forming.

A penile prosthesis or implant is a permanent device that is placed into the penis. Several types of penile prostheses exist that vary in their complexity. There are semirigid prostheses and inflatable prostheses. The semirigid prosthesis remains the same width at all times; you bend the penis up when you wish to have intercourse and down to conceal the penis. This prosthesis is the easiest to put in and has the least risk of mechanical malfunction, but it provides the least natural-looking result. Inflatable prostheses have the advantage of looking natural: in the deflated state, the penis is flaccid, and in the inflated state, the penis becomes erect. Two types of inflatable prostheses are available: a two piece and a three piece. The two-piece unit is composed of two cylinders, one placed in each side of the penis, and a small pump that is placed in the scrotum. Squeezing the scrotal pump pushes fluid into the cylinders, distending them and making the penis erect. The three-piece unit has two cylinders, a scrotal pump, and a reservoir that sits under the abdominal wall near the bladder (**Figure 20**). The reservoir contains a larger amount of fluid, which allows for more rigidity than is possible with the two-piece unit.

As the complexity of the prostheses increases, so does the risk of mechanical trouble. Over the years, these devices have been revised such that the malfunction rate is about 10% at ten years. One of the most distressing risks of placement of a penile prosthesis is infection. Although this risk is small, if the device becomes infected, the whole device must be removed and, in most cases, another device cannot be inserted at the same time. Once a prosthesis has been placed, other forms of treatment for erectile dysfunction usually do not work, although, occasionally, the vacuum device does work in men who have had the prosthesis removed. Thus, it is important to try other forms of therapy for erectile dysfunction and to make sure that they are either ineffective or that you do not like them before you proceed with a penile prosthesis. The satisfaction rate with a penile prosthesis is about 90% for both the man and his partner.

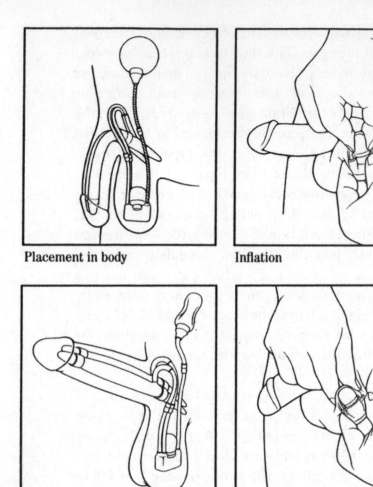

Placement in body

Inflation

Erect state

Deflation

Figure 20 Three-piece penile prosthesis.
Drawings of the AMS 700CX/CXM Penile Prosthesis courtesy of American Medical Systems, Inc., Minnetonka, Minnesota (www.visitAMS.com).

Sural nerve grafting is an investigational therapy for the treatment of erectile dysfunction related to non–nerve sparing radical prostatectomy. During a radical prostatectomy in which the neurovascular bundle(s) are removed, a segment of the sural nerve (a nerve located in the leg) is removed and is sewn into the place where the neurovascular bundle was. Preliminary results with this technique demonstrate that it can improve postoperative erectile dysfunction and that it may also allow for fewer positive margins because the surgeon is able to remove more tissue surrounding the prostate.

Several forms of injection therapy are being evaluated either alone or in combination with PGE-1.

Lastly, a topical gel composed of prostaglandin E1 is being evaluated. This agent would be applied to the penis, and certain chemicals, skin penetration enhancers, would allow the prostaglandin to penetrate through the skin and pass into the corpora to increase penile blood flow.

92. I am incontinent after my prostate cancer. What can I do?

Urinary incontinence, the uncontrolled loss of urine, is one of the most bothersome risks of prostate cancer treatment. Although it is more commonly associated with radical prostatectomy, it may also occur after interstitial seed therapy, EBRT, and cryotherapy. Urinary incontinence may lead to anxiety, hopelessness, and loss of self-control and self-esteem. Fear of leakage may limit social activities and participation in sex. If you are experiencing these feelings, you should discuss this with your doctor and spouse or significant other.

If you experience persistent urinary incontinence after surgery or radiation therapy, your doctor will want to identify the degree and the type of incontinence. You will be asked questions regarding the number of pads you use per day, what activities precipitate the incontinence, how frequently you urinate, if you have frequency or urgency, how strong your force of urine stream is, if you feel that you are emptying your bladder well, and what types and how much fluid you are drinking. The doctor may check to make sure that you are emptying your bladder well. This is usually done by having you urinate and then scanning your bladder with a small ultrasound probe to determine how much urine is left behind. Normally, less than 30 cc (one tablespoon) remains after urination.

Several different types of urinary incontinence exist, and the different types may co-exist. The treatment of urinary incontinence varies with the type, and the types that may be encountered in men being treated for prostate cancer include stress, overflow, and urge incontinence. Men who have undergone radical prostatectomy typically experience a type of stress incontinence called "intrinsic sphincter deficiency." Stress incontinence may also occur after interstitial seed therapy and is much more common if a TURP of the prostate was performed in the past. In men, urinary control is primarily at the bladder outlet by the internal sphincter muscle. This muscle remains closed and opens only during urination. An additional muscle, the external sphincter, is located further away from the bladder and is the "back-up" muscle. The external sphincter is the muscle that you contract when you feel the urge to urinate and there is no bathroom in sight. During a radical prostatectomy, the internal sphincter is often damaged with removal of the prostate because it lies just at the top of the prostate. Continence then depends on the ability of the remaining urethra to close (**coapt**) and on the external sphincter.

Urge incontinence is the involuntary loss of urine associated with the urge to urinate and is related to an overactive bladder. Although less common than intrinsic sphincter deficiency in men who have undergone radical

Coapt

To close or fasten together.

Urge incontinence

The involuntary loss of urine associated with the urge to urinate and is related to an overactive bladder.

prostatectomy, it may be present alone or in conjunction with intrinsic sphincter deficiency. Overactive bladder and decreased bladder capacity are more common in men who have undergone EBRT for prostate cancer.

Overflow incontinence is the involuntary loss of urine related to incomplete emptying of the bladder. After radical prostatectomy, this may occur if significant scarring (a bladder neck contracture) is present at the bladder outlet area. Treatment of the bladder neck contracture often relieves the overflow incontinence. Other symptoms include a weak urine stream and the feeling of incomplete bladder emptying. With overflow incontinence, the bladder scanner would demonstrate a large amount of urine left in the bladder after urinating. Urethral strictures after EBRT may also cause overflow incontinence; dilation of such strictures also improves the overflow incontinence. Urethral strictures tend to recur, and daily in-and-out passage of a catheter beyond the site of the stricture helps prevent recurrence of the stricture. Swelling of the prostate after interstitial seed therapy may cause voiding troubles, which if unrecognized, may lead to overflow incontinence. Initial treatment of overflow incontinence after seed therapy is with clean intermittent catheterization, and possibly the addition of an alpha-blocker and a nonsteroidal anti-inflammatory.

Overflow incontinence

The involuntary loss of urine related to incomplete emptying of the bladder.

Your responses to the questions your doctor asks regarding your incontinence will help your doctor determine the type and the severity of your urinary incontinence. The best way to delineate the type(s) of urinary incontinence that you have is to perform a fluoroscopic urodynamic study, which is a special study designed to measure the pressures in your bladder during voiding and at the time of urinary leakage (if it occurs during the study) and to look at the urethra and bladder during bladder filling and urinating. The study involves the placement of a catheter through the penis into the bladder. The catheter is connected to a pressure monitor, and sterile contrast fluid is run through the catheter into the bladder. Periodic X-ray studies are taken to determine whether the bladder outlet is open and if leakage is occurring. During the study, you will be asked to bear down as though you were trying to have a bowel movement, and you will be checked for leakage during this maneuver. Often, men with **stress incontinence** leak during the bearing down (Valsalva), and the bladder pressure at which this leakage occurs, the Valsalva leak point pressure, is an important predictor of the success of various treatment options. During the urodynamic study, an overactive bladder is identified by intermittent increases in bladder pressure during bladder filling that may be associated with leakage or the urge to urinate.

Stress incontinence

The involuntary loss of urine during sudden rises in intra-abdominal pressure, e.g., with coughing, laughing, sneezing, or picking up heavy objects.

Treatment Options

Once the cause and the severity of the urinary incontinence has been assessed, you can then embark on treatment. In all cases of incontinence, it is important to make sure that you are voiding regularly, that is, every 3 hours, and avoiding alcohol and caffeinated fluids. Caffeine and alcohol cause the kidneys to make more urine and is a bladder irritant. It may also be helpful to avoid acidic foods and foods with a lot of hot spices because these may also act as bladder irritants.

If a bladder neck contracture is present, treatment may consist of dilation or incision. There is a risk of stress incontinence after incision of a bladder neck contracture. If overflow incontinence occurs after interstitial seed therapy, your doctor may give you a medication called an alpha-blocker (which relaxes the prostate) and an anti-inflammatory drug, and also prescribe clean intermittent catheterization until you are voiding on your own. Usually, voiding troubles of this nature after interstitial seed therapy resolve with time; rarely is additional treatment needed. Your doctor will be quite reluctant to do anything more aggressive for the first six months after the placement of the seeds because of the high risk of urinary incontinence with a TURP.

Overactive bladder is treated with medications that relax the bladder muscle, the most common of which are called anticholinergics. Side effects of these medications include dry mouth, facial flushing, constipation, and blurry vision. These are decreased with the long-acting forms.

A variety of treatment options exist for stress incontinence, including Kegel exercises, a penile clamp, collagen injection, an artificial sphincter, a gracilis muscle flap, and a male urethral sling.

- **Pelvic floor muscle exercises**: Pelvic floor muscle exercises are intended to strengthen the pelvic floor muscles. To identify these muscles, simply try stopping your urine stream while you are urinating. These exercises involve repetitive contracting and relaxing of the pelvic muscles at least 20 times per day every day of the week. Pelvic floor stimulation and biofeedback allow you to identify these muscles better and to monitor the strength of the contractions. These exercises are very helpful initially, when the catheter is removed after radical prostatectomy. They are not as effective in men who have undergone prior pelvic irradiation.

- **Penile clamp**: Several penile clamps are available, and all of them have the same principle—to compress the urethra to prevent urinary leakage (**Figure 21**). They should be worn for brief periods of time only and should not be left on all day. If they are left on

Pelvic floor muscle exercises

Exercises that help one strengthen muscles that aid in the control of urinary incontinence.

Penile clamp

A device placed around the penis to prevent urine leakage.

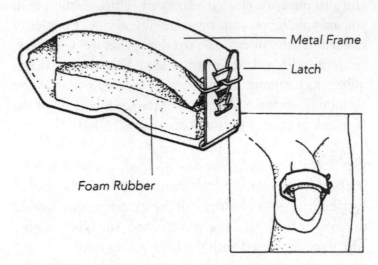

Metal Frame

Latch

Foam Rubber

Figure 21 Penile clamp.
Reprinted by permission of Perseus Books Publishers, a member of Perseus Books LLC.

for long periods of time, they may cause damage to the penile skin and the urethra. The clamp needs to be removed if you need to urinate. The penile clamp should not take the place of Kegel exercises; rather, it should be used as a backup measure, for instance, if you are going out to dinner and want to make certain there is no leakage.

Collagen injection
Artificial urinary sphincter. A prosthesis designed to restore continence in an incontinent person by constricting the urethra.

• **Collagen injection**: Collagen is a chemical that is found throughout your body. The collagen that is being used to treat urinary incontinence is derived from a cow. Because it comes from a source outside of your body, you must have skin testing to make sure that you are not allergic to the collagen. Skin testing involves injecting a small amount of the collagen under your skin and then periodically inspecting the site, as one does with a PPD (tuberculosis) test. If the site becomes red and swollen, then you are allergic to the collagen and cannot undergo collagen injections. However, allergic reactions to collagen are very uncommon.

The collagen is injected into the bladder neck and the proximal urethra to make the urethra come together (coapt) (**Figure 22**). The amount of collagen injected at each treatment varies from person to person. The collagen injection can be performed in the urologist's office under local anesthesia or in the operating room under spinal or general anesthesia. More commonly, the collagen is

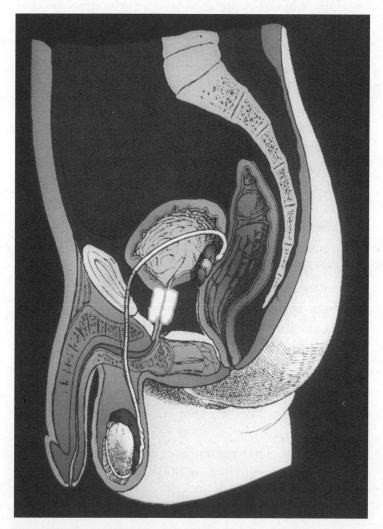

Figure 22 Location of collagen injection.
Courtesy of American Medical Systems, Inc., Minnetonka, Minnesota (www.visitAMS.com).

injected "retrograde" through a cystoscope that is placed through the penile urethra and positioned just before the injection site. A long, thin needle is then passed through the scope and advanced into the urethra at the appropriate location, and the collagen is injected. The collagen is injected at several sites in the urethra until the urologist is satisfied with the amount of urethral coaptation.

Some urologists prefer to perform the procedure antegrade, in which a small needle is passed through the lower abdominal skin into the bladder. A small wire is then placed through the needle into the bladder, and the needle is removed. Small dilators are then placed over the wire to make an opening that is large enough for the cystoscope, which is then placed through the opening in the abdominal skin into the bladder. The bladder neck is identified and the collagen injected. Often, more than one treatment session is needed; typically three to four injections, each four weeks apart, are necessary. It is also possible that repeat collagen injections will be necessary over the long term. Collagen injections provide a continence rate of about 26% in postprostatectomy incontinence and a reduction in the number of pads used per day in an additional 37% of men.

The advantages of collagen injection are that it is minimally invasive, it is repeatable, it is associated with a short recovery period, and if it fails, it does not prevent you from pursuing other forms of therapy. Disadvantages of collagen therapy are that only a small percentage of men become totally dry, a small number of men develop a urinary tract infection, and 11% of men have transient urinary retention requiring clean intermittent catheterization. Permanent retention has not been reported.

Lastly, some individuals will experience transient dysuria (discomfort with voiding) and urgency after the procedure. The best candidates for collagen are men who have higher Valsalva leak point pressures (> 60 cm H_2O), who do not have overactive bladders, have not had prior radiation or cryotherapy, and who have not had a vigorous incision of a bladder neck contracture.

- **Artificial urinary sphincter**: The artificial sphincter is a mechanical device that is composed of a cuff that is placed around the urethra, a pump that is placed in the scrotum, and a reservoir that is positioned in the abdomen (**Figures 23** and **24**). All of these parts and the tubing that connects them are buried under the skin and are not visible. The cuff remains filled with sterile fluid and compresses the urethra. When you wish to urinate, the pump is pressed, and this transfers fluid out of the cuff, allowing you to urinate. The cuff automatically refills to compress the urethra. Placement of the artificial sphincter requires general or spinal anesthesia and an overnight hospital stay. Initially after the surgery, the sphincter is "deactivated" so that it doesn't work. It will be "activated" 4 to 6 weeks after surgery, when the tissues have healed and the swelling and sensitivity have subsided. The artificial sphincter provides continence rates of 20% to 90%, including men who are either totally dry or who use one pad per day. The sphincter can be used after collagen has failed. Disadvantages of the sphincter include mechanical malfunction rates of 10 to 15%, erosion rates of zero to 5%, and infection rates of 3%. Erosion is the migration of the device into another site. The cuff may erode into the urethra or through the skin, and other

Artificial urinary sphincter

A prosthesis designed to restore continence in an incontinent person by constricting the urethra.

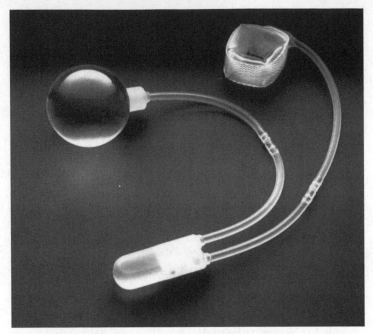

Figure 23 AMS Sphincter 800 urinary prosthesis.
Courtesy of American Medical Systems, Inc., Minnetonka, Minnesota (www.visitAMS.com).

parts of the sphincter may erode into the skin or other areas. If there is an erosion, the device must be removed. Similarly, if the sphincter becomes infected, it must be removed. It is very important that a urodynamic study be performed before the sphincter is placed to make sure that the bladder holds an adequate amount of urine at low pressures and to identify an overactive bladder, which would require additional treatment.

Gracilis myoplasty

A surgical procedure whereby a muscle in the leg, the gracilis muscle, is repositioned around the urethra.

- **Gracilis myoplasty**: Gracilis myoplasty is a surgical procedure whereby a muscle in the leg is repositioned around the urethra, like the cuff of the artificial sphincter. Thus, it acts as a natural cuff. This procedure is performed in only a small number of institutions throughout the country and is not used as a first line of treatment. Rather, it

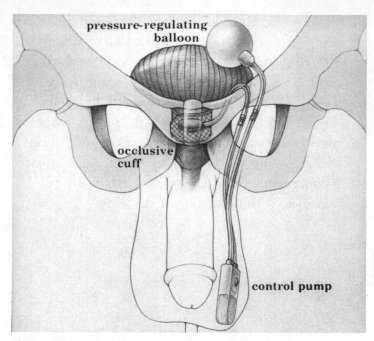

Figure 24 Location of artificial sphincter.

AMS sphincter 800 urinary prothesis courtesy of American Medical Systems, Inc., Minnetonka, Minnesota (www.visitAMS.com).

may have a role in men who have had prior radiation therapy or cryotherapy and for those in whom an artificial sphincter was removed for cuff erosion.

- **Male sling**: The fascial sling has been used for several years in women with stress incontinence and has proved to be a successful and durable procedure. Because of its success in women, it has been used more recently in men who are incontinent after radical prostatectomy. The sling may be derived from the patient's own tissues, from a synthetic (manmade) material, or from cadavers. The goal of the sling is to place tissue under the urethra to act as a buttress or a hammock. The tissue is anchored to either the abdominal wall or the pubic bone.

Male sling

A procedure to promote urinary continence in which a piece of tissue is placed under the urethra to act as a hammock or buttress.

Because this procedure is new, the long-term success rate is not known. Over the short term, about 50% of men become dry, and an additional 8% experience improvement in their incontinence. This is a surgical procedure that usually involves an overnight stay in the hospital. Urinary retention may occur that requires CIC over the short term and loosening of the sling if persistent. Persistent incontinence after the sling is inserted may be improved with tightening of the sling.

PART SEVEN

Social Effects of Prostate Cancer

I don't have a job or insurance. How can I get my prostate checked?

Are there support groups for men with prostate cancer, and if so, how do I find out about these?

I've never thought of dying before, but now that I have been diagnosed with prostate cancer, I think about it and wonder if there are things that I should be doing to prepare myself for the inevitable.

More . . .

93. I don't have a job or insurance. How can I get my prostate checked?

In the fall, Prostate Cancer Awareness Week typically includes free prostate cancer screening. This screening includes a digital rectal examination and a PSA level determination. The examining physician tells you whether he or she thinks your prostate feels suspicious and whether further evaluation by a urologist is recommended. You receive your PSA results by mail at a later time. If your PSA is elevated, you will be told that further evaluation is indicated, and you will be expected to make an appointment with a urologist for this. Often, this service is provided at your local hospital and may be advertised in the newspaper. If you have not seen advertisements in the past, you may want to call your local hospital(s) to see if it is offered. If you are not able to obtain any information from your local hospital, you may want to try the offices of local urologists. If you plan to return to the free prostate cancer screening on a yearly basis, keep in mind that the same person may not examine your prostate each year and the PSA results from year to year may not be compared. For this reason, it is important that you keep track of the results and compare them yourself. Ideally, the PSA should not change by more than 0.7 to 0.75 ng/mL per year, even if each of the values is within the normal range. If the change is greater than 0.7 ng/mL per year, even if both numbers fall within the "normal range," then you should seek further evaluation. Transrectal ultrasound–guided prostate biopsies are not part of the free prostate cancer screening.

94. Are there support groups for men with prostate cancer, and if so, how do I find out about these?

Yes, there are prostate cancer support groups. These often can be found at your local hospital and meet on a regular basis. At our institution, they are held on a monthly basis. Often, there are guest speakers at the support groups to address key concerns of the group, such as nutrition, treatment of erectile dysfunction, treatment of urinary incontinence, and updates on newer forms of chemotherapy, in addition to group discussion time. Prostate cancer support groups provide an informal setting to express one's concerns, ask questions, and share information with others. Often, spouses and significant others attend and are invited to discuss their concerns. Discussing some of your concerns with others who are going or have gone through what you are experiencing may help alleviate some of your anxieties and help you focus on what questions you need to have answered by your doctor(s) as you make treatment decisions. To find out about your local prostate cancer support group, ask your urologist or your local hospital. The American Cancer Society (see Appendix) may also be able to help you identify a local prostate cancer support group.

95. I've never thought of dying before, but now that I have been diagnosed with prostate cancer, I think about it and wonder if there are things that I should be doing to prepare myself for the inevitable.

None of us like to think about our life ending, particularly if we feel healthy. Because we don't like to think about dying, we often do not prepare for it. All individuals, whether they are healthy or ill, need to think about death. End-of-life decisions, such as one's views on resuscitation measures and living wills, should be addressed long before one becomes ill. Financial issues and wills should be prepared and discussed with your family in advance. There is nothing more disheartening than for someone to become ill and not be able to make decisions, leaving the family at a loss as to what that individual would want. This is extremely important for measures like resuscitation, in the event that your heart stops, and other interventions to prolong life, such as nutritional support and ventilatory support (breathing machines). In addition, if you are in charge of the finances, it is important for you to identify one family member to discuss financial matters with early so that you may counsel that person as to how to manage the finances in your absence.

If you are unclear about what legal issues need to be addressed, it may be helpful to consult a lawyer. The American Cancer Society has a brochure that discusses more common things that need to be addressed, including questions regarding business, taxes, and loans. You will want to make sure that the following are in order and that you discuss them in advance with your family: life insurance, retirement plans, titles to assets, property, bank accounts, debts, safe deposit boxes, stock, car deeds, and will. It is important that beneficiaries are designated and that account numbers, addresses, telephone numbers, and contact people are recorded. All of this information is in a location that is accessible to your family, and your family needs to know that you have taken care of these matters.

96. How will treatment of my prostate cancer affect my sexuality?

All forms of treatment of prostate cancer, with the exception of watchful waiting, have the risk of causing erectile dysfunction. Hormone therapy affects libido (desire for sex) in addition to erection function. But erectile function is only one part of your overall sexual function, and other phases of your sexual response can occur without a rigid penis. Sexual arousal can occur with other forms of stimulation and does not require penile rigidity. Orgasm also occurs in the absence of penile rigidity. After a radical prostatectomy, you have a dry ejaculate (no fluid will come out of the penis). The ejaculate volume may also be affected to varying degrees by interstitial seed therapy and EBRT.

It is very important to realize that your "sexuality" and your partner's sexual fulfillment are not lost because you can't achieve a rigid erection. Should you choose not to proceed with treatment for erectile dysfunction, you and your spouse or partner can still have a fulfilling sex life. It may require that you both re-address your own sensuality and what is stimulating for each of you and incorporate this into your sexual life. Thus, what is so often perceived as a "devastating" side effect of prostate cancer treatment can actually bring you and your spouse or partner closer together if both of you are willing to openly discuss sexual preferences, other forms of stimulation, and so on. Studies have demonstrated that many men are concerned that when they lose their erectile function, they are no longer a "man." On the contrary, women indicate that, in general, they do not think that this causes their spouse or husband to be any less of a man, and they indicate that other forms of intimacy, such as hugging, touching, and kissing, are just as important to them as sexual intercourse. Lastly, many women find that they are better able to achieve an orgasm with touching and finger stimulation than with vaginal intercourse.

Retreating and avoiding sex may only cause you more stress and anxiety. If you find it hard to discuss your sexuality and the changes that have occurred, then it may be helpful to seek out a specialist who can help you and your spouse adjust to the changes that have occurred in a more positive manner.

97. I've just found out that I have prostate cancer and I am depressed. Is this common?

Cliff's comment:

When you get the news, especially when there have been no warning signs and you are feeling great—to say that you may get depressed is an understatement. I had just recently retired, bought a beautiful home on a lake, and was looking forward to so many things; then I was told I have that horrible thing, CANCER. I became very anxious and depressed. My wife begged me to get some temporary medication while I was waiting to undergo the radical prostatectomy, but I refused. I was "too strong of a man" for that stuff—BIG MISTAKE! In the time it took for the results of my prostate biopsy to return and for me to undergo the radical prostatectomy, my blood pressure climbed significantly as a result of my anxieties. Instead of treating the underlying problem, I was given higher and higher doses of blood pressure medications. Well, that didn't help me and may have contributed to some of my problems in the postoperative period. Next time, I'll listen to my wife. An antidepressant to help me get through those few weeks before surgery would have been very helpful for me—I was a wreck, and it would have been nice to have had the help.

The diagnosis of prostate cancer comes as a shock to most men. Often, they are feeling fine and experience no signs or symptoms to make them suspicious. When they are faced with such a shock, common reactions are fear, anger, confusion, and depression. It is not unusual to initially "retreat" from life as you absorb the reality of the situation and begin to gather information and start the decision-making process. If you find that you have feelings of failure, are continuing to withdraw socially, feel that you are being punished, are thinking about committing suicide, feel helpless and can't make decisions, have lost interest in activities that brought you pleasure, or are crying a lot, then you may suffer from a more severe depression and you should discuss this with your doctor. Sometimes, when faced with such potentially overwhelming situations, you may need some assistance to help you gain control of your life again and make the decisions you will need to make regarding your treatment.

98. How will the diagnosis of prostate cancer affect me, my spouse/partner, and our relationship?

Cliff's comment:

I had just recently retired, bought a dream house on the water, and was thinking about the future. Finding out that I had prostate cancer and the acute realization that perhaps I did not have too long to live made me look critically at my future and my relationship with my family. Looking back, I realize how supportive my wife and family were throughout the whole ordeal. My wife helped me get over the initial shock, got me through the surgical recovery, and kept me thinking optimistically as I waited for my first PSA value after the surgery. My children also rallied on my behalf. My son stayed with me several nights in the hospital, which I realize must have been very difficult for him, as he is aware that he is at increased risk for prostate cancer.

I thank God each day for the blessing that he has bestowed on me. I live each day to the fullest. I am no longer putting things off to the future. I am very thankful that I will continue to be able to see my grandchildren grow up, and I take advantage of each opportunity that I have to be with my family. I feel that the stresses that I went through both before and after surgery and my family's support during this time have brought us all closer together.

Each individual is different, and each relationship is different, so it is hard to generalize about how each of you, and the two of you together, will react. In general, it appears that there are different aspects of prostate cancer and its treatment that are more stressful for you and your spouse or partner. Men generally appear to be most concerned with changes that are related to the treatment of prostate cancer, namely erectile dysfunction and urinary incontinence. Women, however, are more concerned about long-term survival. It appears that as couples face the challenge of dealing with prostate cancer, one of the critical steps is re-establishing their commitment to each other. This is achieved by open communication, which may be verbal or nonverbal, such as a hug. The absence of this sense of reconnection between partners, often as a result of failure of communication, can distance the relationship and make mutual support more difficult.

There is a delicate balance for couples between acknowledging fears that arise and keeping them private. Either extreme, being too vocal or too private, appears to create tension. Sometimes men do not express their worries and fears because they are concerned about the effect that this may have on their spouse. They often indicate that they have held things back because they didn't want to worry their spouses or felt that their spouses were not strong enough to deal with the issues. It is important that you communicate your concerns and fears with someone, whether it be your physician, close friend, relative, or men going through similar experiences, if you feel that you cannot discuss them with your spouse or significant other. Prostate cancer support groups, such as "Man to Man" or "Us Too," may be very helpful in this situation.

Confronting a life-threatening illness is difficult, but through open communication and mutual support, it can draw a family closer together, force a reordering of priorities, and influence a change toward a healthier lifestyle for all of those affected.

99. My husband/partner was just diagnosed with prostate cancer. What can I do to help him?

The diagnosis of prostate cancer can be devastating. Initially, shock and sadness are present, then once the shock has worn off, the decision-making process begins. Most men need to re-establish equilibrium, to get things back in order, as soon as possible. Taking an active role in the decision-making process tends to alleviate some of their anxieties. Men tend to be less vocal about their concerns and worries than women; whereas women tend to confide their concerns and worries to close friends and relatives, men often share this information only with their spouse or partner. You are indeed your husband's/partner's main, possibly only, support system, and this is very important to him. Your support, reassurance, and efforts in helping him acknowledge and cope with the diagnosis and treatment of prostate cancer will encourage him considerably. Studies have shown that married men with prostate cancer live longer than divorced, widowed, or single men with prostate cancer. It appears that this is related to the emotional support and possibly better health habits that married men have. Thus, helping your husband or partner maintain or optimize his health can be very important. Proper nutrition (see Question 17) and physical exercise will be of great benefit from both a physical and an emotional standpoint.

It is important to periodically reaffirm your commitment to the relationship and your partner/husband. Your awareness of your husband or partner's need to return to normal life as soon as possible and your willingness to facilitate this will help him greatly. Supporting your husband's efforts to seek help if he is feeling despondent and depressed is also important.

100. Will I be able to do the things I used to do now that I have prostate cancer? Can I travel? Can I golf?

Cliff's comment:

Since I had my radical prostatectomy, I can enjoy all of the things that I could before surgery. I am golfing and hiking and feel like my previous self. The only recognizable limitation that I am aware of now is that I cannot donate blood at this time—I must be a cancer survivor for five years before they will accept my blood. In January 2004, I will happily arrive at the local Red Cross facility and gladly donate a pint of blood to help someone else.

All forms of therapy may fatigue you for a few weeks after the procedure, but by one month after treatment, you should be back to full activity.

A lot of what you will be able to do will vary with the stage of your disease and the treatment that you are undergoing. With early-stage prostate cancer, there are usually few limitations; you can golf, travel, and so on. If you are planning to undergo surgical treatment, you will want to take good care of yourself before surgery. It is helpful to make sure that you are eating right, resting, and getting regular exercise.

There will be a recovery period after the surgery, and your doctor will indicate when he or she feels that you can resume full activity. The recovery period varies with the surgical procedure used. Recovery from the laparoscopic approach appears to be quicker than with the traditional open approach, and with interstitial seed therapy, the convalescence is much shorter than with surgery. If, however, you have trouble voiding after the procedure, you may require clean intermittent catheterization until the swelling in your prostate subsides. You can travel while performing clean intermittent catheterization; you just need to pack a catheter and the lubricating jelly. Radiation therapy takes several weeks to complete, and because it is performed 5 of the 7 days of the week, it requires that you "stay put" for a period of time. All forms of therapy may fatigue you for a few weeks after the procedure, but by one month after treatment, you should be back to full activity. If you are receiving the intramuscular form of hormone therapy and you wish to travel, you can make arrangements with urologists in the area to which you are traveling to get the shots. Often, your doctor can send a letter to the urologist in advance.

There are many organizations and publications that can provide you with more information. A list of many such resources is provided in the Appendix.

Appendix

Organizations

American Academy of Medical Acupuncture
www.medicalacupuncture.org
By Telephone: 323-937-5514
By Mail: AAMA, 4929 Wilshire Boulevard, Suite 428, Los Angeles,
California 90010

American Cancer Society
www.cancer.org
By Telephone: 1-800-ACS-2345
By Mail: American Cancer Society National Home Office, 1599 Clifton Road,
Atlanta, GA 30329
American Cancer Society Man to Man Support Groups
www.cancer.org/docroot/CRI/content/

American Foundation For Urologic Disease/Prostate Health Council
www.afud.org
By Telephone: 800-242-2383
By Mail: 300 West Pratt Street, Suite 401, Baltimore, MD 21201-2463

American Prostate Society
www.ameripros.org
By Telephone: 410-859-3735
By Fax: 410-850-0818
By Mail: 1340-F Charwood Rd, Hanover, MD 21076

American Society of Clinical Oncology
www.asco.org
By Telephone: 703-299-0150
By Mail: 1900 Duke Street, Suite 200, Alexandria, VA 22314

American Urological Association
www.AUAnet.org—clinical guidelines for the management of locally confined
prostate cancer 2007 guidelines

American Urological Association Foundation
Patient Education 1000 Corporate Boulevard Linthicum,
MD 21090 Toll Free (U.S. only): 1-866-RING AUA
(1-866-746-4282)
Phone: 410-689-3700
Fax: 410-689-3800
www.auafoundation.org   www.urology health.org

Cancer Care, Inc.
www.cancercare.org
By Telephone: 212-712-8400 (admin); 212-712-8080 (services)
By Mail: 275 7th Avenue, New York, NY 10001

Cancer Research Institute
www.cancerresearch.org
By Telephone: 1-800-99-CANCER (800-992-26237)
By Mail: Cancer Research Institute, 681 Fifth Avenue,
New York, NY 10022

**CaPcure (The Association for the Cure of Cancer
   of the Prostate)**
www.capcure.org
By Telephone: 800-757-CURE or 310-458-2873
By Mail: 1250 4th Street, Santa Monica, CA 90401

Centers for Disease Control and Prevention (CDC)
www.cdc.gov
By Telephone: 404-639-3534
Toll Free Number: 800-311-3435
By Mail: Centers for Disease Control and Prevention, 1600
Clifton Rd., Atlanta, GA 30333

Department of Veterans Affairs
www.va.gov
By Telephone: 202-273-5400 (Washington, D.C. office)
Toll Free Number: 800-827-1000 (reaches local VA office)
By Mail: Veterans Health Association, 810 Vermont Ave., NW,
Washington, DC, 20420

Health Insurance Association of America (HIAA)
www.hiaa.org
By Telephone: 202-824-1600
By Mail: 555 13th Street NW, Suite 600, East Washington,
D.C. 20004-1109

Health Resources and Services Administration
Hill-Burton Program
www.hrsa.gov/osp/dfcr/about/aboutdiv.htm
By Telephone: 301-443-5656
Toll Free Number: 800-638-0742
                    800-492-0359 (if calling from the Maryland area)
By Mail: Health Resources and Services Administration,
U.S. Department of Health and Human Services,
Parklawn Building, 5600 Fishers Lane, Rockville, MD 20857

International Cancer Alliance (ICARE)
www.icare.org/icare
By Telephone: 800-ICARE-61 or 301-654-7933
By Mail: 4853 Cordell Avenue, Suite 11, Bethesda, MD 20814
By Fax: 201-654-8684

National Cancer Institute
www.nci.nih.gov
By Telephone: 301-435-3848 (Public Information Office line)
By Mail: National Cancer Institute Public Information Office,
Building 31, Room 10A31, 31 Center Drive, MSC 2580,
Bethesda, Maryland 20892-2580

National Center for Complementary and Alternative Medicine
nccam.nih.gov
By Telephone: 1-888-644-6226
By Mail: NCCAM Clearinghouse, P.O. Box 7923,
Gaithersburg, Maryland 20898

National Comprehensive Cancer Network
www.nccn.org
By Telephone: 888-909-NCCN (888-909-6226)
By Mail: National Comprehensive Cancer Network,
50 Huntingdon Pike, Suite 200, Rockledge, PA 19046

Prostate Cancer

Astra Zeneca Pharmaceuticals LP
www.prostateinfo.com

The Prostate Cancer Education Council
By Telephone: 800-813-HOPE, 212-302-2400
By Mail: 1180 Avenue of the Americas, New York, NY 10036

The Prostate Cancer Infolink
www.comed.com/prostate
By Mail: c/o CoMed Communications, Inc., 210 West
Washington Square, Philadelphia, PA 19106

Prostate Cancer Research and Education Foundation
 (PC-REF)
www.prostatecancer.com
By Telephone: 619-287-8860
By Fax: 619-287-8890
By Mail: 6699 Alvaro Rd, Suite 2301, San Diego, CA 92120

Prostate Cancer Resource Network
pcrn.org
By Telephone: 800-915-1001 or 813-848-2494
By Fax: 813-847-1619
By Mail: P.O. Box 966, Newport Richey, FL 34656

Social Security Administration
Office of Public Inquiries
www.ssa.gov
By Telephone: 800-772-1213
                  800-325-0778 (TTY)
By Mail: Social Security Administration, Office of Public
Inquiries, 6401 Security Blvd., Room 4-C-5 Annex, Baltimore,
MD 21235-6401

United Seniors Health Cooperative (USHC)
www.unitedseniorshealth.org
By Telephone: 202-479-6973
Toll Free Number: 800-637-2604
By Mail: USHC, Suite 200, 409 Third St, SW,
Washington, DC 20024

US TOO International, Inc.
www.ustoo.com
By Telephone: 800-808-7866, 630-323-1002
By Fax: 630-323-1003
By Mail: 903 North York Rd, Suite 50, Hinsdale, IL
60521-2993

Web Sites with General Cancer Information

411Cancer.com
About.com (search on "cancer")
CancerLinks.org
CancerSource.com
CancerWiseTM/MD Anderson Cancer Center,
    www.cancerwise.org
National Cancer Institute's CancerNet Service,
    cancernet.nci.nih.gov/index.html.

Web Pages on Specific Topics

Alternative Therapy
Information on acupuncture: www.medicalacupuncture.org
(see American Academy for Medical Acupuncture)

Comprehensive web site about alternative therapies for cancer:
www.healthy.net/asp/templates/center.asp?centerid=23

Chemotherapy
www.yana.org offers online and in-person support groups for
those going through high-dose chemotherapy.

Drug information for chemotherapy and hormonal therapy,
including information on financial assistance:
www.cancersupportivecare.com/pharmacy.html.

Clinical Trials
National Cancer Institute's CancerTrials site lists current clinical
trials that have been reviewed by NCI.

Coping

National Coalition for Cancer Survivorship (www.cansearch.org, 877-NCCS-YES) offers a free audio program, "Cancer Survivor Toolbox, including ways to cope with the illness. (Web site also has a newsletter, requiring yearly membership fee)

R. A. Bloch Cancer Foundation (www.blochcancer.org) offers an inspirational online book about cancer, relaxation techniques, and positive outlooks on fighting cancer, as well as trained one-onone support from fellow cancer patients.

Diet and Nutrition (Cancer Prevention)

USDA Dietary Guidelines: www.usda.gov/cnpp

American Institute for Cancer Research provides tips on how to reduce cancer risk. www.aicr.org

Cancer Research Foundation of America's Healthy Eating Suggestions: www.preventcancer.org/whdiet.cfm

Family Resources

www.kidscope.org is a website designed to help children understand and deal with the effects of cancer on a parent

Genetic Counseling

The National Society of Genetic Counselors web site (www.nsgc.org) lists society members, complete with specialty.

The National Cancer Institute has a searchable list of health care professionals who specialize in genetics and can provide information and counseling. http://cancernet.nci.nih.gov/genesrch.shtml

Articles on genetics and cancer:
http://cancer.med.upenn.edu/causeprevent/genetics

Legal Protections, Financial Resources, and Insurance Coverage

The American Cancer Society offers a number of relevant documents to help understand your coverage, legal protections, and how to find financial assistance. Search http://www.cancer.org using keyword "insurance."

Medicaid Information:
www.hcfa.gov/medical/medicaid.htm

Family and Medical Leave Act:
www.dol.gov/dol/esa/public/regs/statutes/whd/fmla.htm

Health Care Financing Administration's (HCFA) information
website about Breast Cancer and Medicaid programs:
www.hcfa.gov/medicaid/bccpt/default.htm

www.needymeds.com offers information about programs
sponsored by pharmaceutical manufacturers to help people who
cannot afford to purchase necessary drugs.

www.cancercare.org/hhrd/hhrd_financial.htm offers listings of
where to look for financial assistance.

The National Financial Resource Book for Patients:
A State-by-State Directory: data.patientadvocate.org/

Nausea/Vomiting
National Comprehensive Cancer Network:
www.nccn.org/patient_guidelines/nausea-and-vomiting/
  nausea-and-vomiting/1_introduction.htm

Royal Marsden Hospital Patient Information On Line:
www.royalmarsden.org/patientinfo/booklets/coping/
  nausea7.asp#heading

Treatment Locators: Physicians and Hospitals
AIM DocFinder (*State Medical Board Executive Directors*):
www.docboard.org/

Nonprofit organization providing a health professional licensing
database.

AMA Physician Select (*American Medical Association*):
www.amaassn.org/aps/amahg.htm

AMA database of demographic and professional information on
individual physicians in the United States.

American Board of Medical Specialties: provides verification of
physician qualifications and has lists of specialists.
www.abms.org/, 1-866-ASK-ABMS or American Board of
Medical Specialties, 1007 Church Street, Suite 404,
Evanston, IL 60201-5913

Best Hospitals Finder (*U.S. News & World Report*):
www.usnews.com/usnews/nycu/health/hosptl/tophosp.htm

The *U.S. News* hospital rankings are designed to assist patients
in their search for the highest level of medical care. Database is
searchable by specialty, including the top cancer hospitals
(www.usnews.com/usnews/nycu/health/hosptl/speccanc.htm) or
by geographic region.

Best HMOs Finder (*U.S. News & World Report*):
www.usnews.com/usnews/nycu/health/hetophmo.htm
U.S. News guide to choosing a managed-care option.

Hospital Select (*American Medical Association & Medical-Net,Inc.*):
www.hospitalselect.com/curb_db/owa/sp_hospselect.main

Hospital locator database searchable by hospital name, city,
state, or zip code. Hospital Select data include basic information
(name, address, telephone number); beds and utilization; service
lines; and accreditation.

National Cancer Institute Designated Cancer Centers:
cancertrials.nci.nih.gov/finding/centers/html/map.html

Directory of NCI-designated Cancer Centers, 58 research-
oriented U.S. institutions recognized for scientific excellence
and extensive cancer resources. Listings feature phone contact
numbers, website links and a brief summary of website resources.

National Comprehensive Cancer Network (NCCN):
www.nccn.org

The National Comprehensive Cancer Network (NCCN) is an
alliance of leading cancer centers. NCCN members
(www.nccn.org/profiles.htm) provide the highest quality in
cancer care and cancer research. NCCN offers a patient information and referral service (www.nccn.org/newsletters/1999_may/
page_5.htm) that responds to cancer-related inquiries and
provides referrals to member institutions' programs and services
(1-888-909-6226).

Approved Hospital Cancer Program (*Commission on Cancer of the American College of Surgeons*):
www.facs.org/public_info/yourhealth/aahcp.html

The Approvals Program of the Commission on Cancer surveys hospitals, treatment centers, and other facilities according to standards set by the Committee on Approvals, which recommends approval awards in specific categories based on these surveys.
A hospital that has received approval has voluntarily committed itself to providing the best in diagnosis and treatment of cancer. Approved hospitals can be searched by city, state, and category.

Association of Community Cancer Centers: Cancer Centers and Member Profiles:
www.accc-cancer.org/members/map.html

Geographic listing of ACCC members with contact information, and description of cancer program and services *as provided by the member institutions.*

HMOs and Other Managed Care Plans (Cancer Care):
www.cancercare.org/patients/hmos.htm

Discusses the advantages and disadvantages of HMO care.

Physician Qualifications
The American Board of Medical Specialities www.abms.org; click on "who's certified" button (search by physician name or by specialty)

Radiation Therapy
National Cancer Institute/CancerNet: Radiation Therapy and You: A Guide to Self-Help During Cancer Treatment cancernet.nci.nih.gov/peb/radiation/. By phone, free of charge: 1-800-4-CANCER (in English and Spanish)

Books and Pamphlets

The following pamphlets are available from the National Cancer Institute by calling 1-800-4-CANCER:
- "Chemotherapy and You: A Guide to Self-Help During Treatment"
- "Eating Hints for Cancer Patients Before, During, and After Treatment"

- "Get Relief From Cancer Pain"
- "Helping Yourself During Chemotherapy"
- "Questions and Answers About Pain Control: A Guide for People with Cancer and Their Families"
- "Taking Time: Support for People With Cancer and the People Who Care About Them"
- "Taking Part in Clinical Trials: What Cancer Patients Need to Know"

Available in Spanish:
- "Datos sobre el tratamiento de quimioterapia contra el cancer"
- "El tratamiento de radioterapia; guia para el paciente durante el tratamiento"
- "En que consisten los estudios clinicos? Un folleto para los pacientes de cancer"

The following pamphlets are available from the National Comprehensive Cancer Network:
- *Prostate Cancer Treatment Guidelines for Patients*
- *Cancer Pain Treatment Guidelines for Patients*
- *Nausea and Vomiting Treatment Guidelines for Patient with Cancer*

Available in Spanish:
- *Cáncer de la próstata*
- *El dolor asociado con el cáncer*

Carney KL, 1998. *What is Cancer Anyway? Explaining Cancer to Children of All Ages.*

Hapham WH, 1997. *When a Parent Has Cancer: A Guide to Caring for Your Children.*

Landay, D, 1998. *Be Prepared: The Complete Financial, Legal, and Practical Guide for Living with a Life-challenging Condition.*

Glossary

A

Active surveillance: A form of prostate cancer therapy whereby no definitive treatment is instituted initially, but definitive therapy is instituted when predefined changes are noted.

Abdomen: The part of the body below the ribs and above the pelvic bone that contains organs such as the intestines, the liver, the kidneys, the stomach, the bladder, and the prostate.

Adenocarcinoma: A form of cancer that develops from a malignant abnormality in the cells lining a glandular organ such as the prostate; almost all prostate cancers are adenocarcinomas.

Acupuncture: A Chinese therapy involving the use of thin needles inserted into specific locations in the skin.

Adrenal glands: Glands located above each kidney. These glands produce several different hormones including sex hormones.

Alkaline phosphatase: Chemical (enzyme) that is produced in the liver and bones. It is often elevated when prostate cancer has spread to the bones.

Alternative treatment: The treatment is used instead of accepted treatments.

Androgen blockade: To prevent the effects of the male hormones (androgens).

Androgens: Hormones that are necessary for the development and function of the male sexual organs and male sexual characteristics (i.e., hair, voice change).

Anesthesia: The loss of feeling or sensation: With respect to surgery, means the loss of sensation of pain, as it is induced to allow surgery or other painful procedures to be performed. General: A state of unconsciousness, produced by anesthetic agents, with absence of pain sensation over the entire body and a greater or lesser degree of muscle relaxation. Local: Anesthesia confined to one part of the body. Spinal: Anesthesia produced by injection of a local anesthetic into the subarachnoid space around the spinal cord.

Antiandrogen: A medication that eliminates or reduces the presence or activity of androgens.

Antigen: A substance that stimulates the individual's body to produce cells that fight off the antigen, and in doing so, kill cancer cells.

Antioxidant: A chemical that helps prevent changes in cells and reduce damage to the cell that can cause it to become cancerous.

Anus: The outside opening of the rectum.

Apex of the prostate: The end of the prostate gland located farthest away from the urinary bladder.

Artificial urinary sphincter: A prosthesis designed to restore continence in an incontinent person by constricting the urethra.

B

Benign: A growth that is not cancerous.

Benign prostatic hyperplasia: See BPH.

BID: Twice a day.

Bilateral: Both sides.

Biochemical progression: Recurrence of prostate cancer as defined by an elevation in PSA.

Biopsy: The removal of small sample(s) of tissue for examination under the microscope.

Biphosphonate: A type of medication that is used to treat osteoporosis and the bone pain caused by some types of cancer.

Bladder: The hollow organ that stores and discharges urine from the body.

Bladder catheterization: Passage of a catheter into the urinary bladder to drain urine.

Bladder neck: The outlet area of the bladder. It is composed of circular muscle fibers and helps in the control of urine.

Bladder neck contracture: Scar tissue at the bladder neck that causes narrowing.

Bladder outlet: The first part of the natural channel through which urine passes when it leaves the bladder.

Bladder outlet obstruction: Obstruction of the bladder outlet causing problems with urination and/ or retention of urine in the bladder.

Bladder spasm: A sudden contraction of the bladder, which one is not able to control, that often produces pain and a feeling of the need to urinate.

Bone scan: A specialized nuclear medicine study that allows one to detect changes in the bone that may be related to metastatic prostate cancer.

Bound PSA: PSA attached to the proteins in the bloodstream.

Bowel prep: Cleansing (and sterilization) of the intestines before abdominal surgery.

BPH (benign prostatic hyperplasia): Noncancerous enlargement of the prostate.

Brachytherapy: A form of radiation therapy whereby radioactive pellets are placed into the prostate.

C

Cancer: Abnormal and uncontrolled growth of cells in the body that may spread, injure areas of the body, and lead to death.

Capsule: A fibrous outer layer that surrounds the prostate.

Carcinoma: A form of cancer that originates in tissues that line or cover a particular organ; see adenocarcinoma.

Castration: The removal of both testicles.

Catheter: A hollow tube that allows for fluid drainage from or injection into an area.

Cell: The smallest unit of the body. Tissues in the body are made up of cells.

Chemoprevention: The use of a substance to prevent the development and growth of cancer.

Chemotherapy: A treatment for cancer that uses powerful medications to weaken and destroy the cancer cells.

Chromosome: Part of the cell that carries genes and functions in the transmission of hereditary information.

Clean intermittent catheterization (CIC): The placement of a catheter into the bladder to drain urine and the removal after the urine is drained at defined intervals throughout the day to allow for bladder emptying. It may also be performed to maintain patency after treatment of a bladder neck contracture or urethral stricture.

Clinical trials: A carefully planned experiment to evaluate a treatment or medication (often a new drug) for an unproven use.

Coapt: To close or fasten together.

Collagen injection: A prosthesis designed to restore continence in an incontinent person by constricting the urethra.

Colostomy: A surgical opening between the colon (large intestine) and the skin that allows stool to drain into a collecting bag.

Complementary medicine: A new treatment intended to be used in addition to the standard proven treatment option.

Complication: An undesirable result of a treatment, surgery, or medication.

Conformal EBRT: EBRT that uses CT scan images to better visualize radiation targets and normal tissues.

Contracture: Scarring which can occur at the bladder neck after radical prostatectomy or radiation therapy and result in decreased force of urine stream and incomplete bladder emptying.

Cryotherapy, cryosurgery: A prostate cancer therapy in which the prostate is frozen to destroy the cancer cells.

CT scan/CAT scan (computerized tomography/computerized axial tomography): A specialized X-ray study that allows one to visualize internal structures in cross-section to look for abnormalities.

Cystoscope: A telescope-like instrument that allows one to examine the urethra and inside of the bladder.

Cystoscopy: The procedure of using a cystoscope to look into the urethra and bladder.

D

Debulk: To decrease the amount of cancer present by surgery, hormone therapy, or chemotherapy.

Deep venous thrombosis (DVT): The formation of a blood clot in the large deep veins, usually of the legs or in the pelvis.

Deferred therapy: Delaying treatment until the cancer appears to be a threat to the patient.

Dihydrotestosterone (DHT): A breakdown product of testosterone, which is more powerful than testosterone.

Diagnosis: The identification of the cause or presence of a medical problem or disease.

Digital rectal examination (DRE): The examination of the prostate by placing a gloved finger into the rectum.

Disease: Any change from or interruption of the normal structure or function of any part, organ, system of the body that presents with characteristic symptoms and signs, and whose cause and prognosis may be known or unknown.

Dissection: The surgical removal of tissue.

Double-blind: A research study in which neither the patient nor the doctor (investigator) knows what medication the patient is taking.

Doubling time: The amount of time that it takes for the cancer to double in size.

Down-size: To shrink or reduce the size of the cancer.

Down-stage: To reduce the initial stage of the cancer to a lower (better prognostic) stage.

E

Early prostate cancer antigen: see EPCA.

Ejaculation: The release of semen through the penis during orgasm: After radical prostatectomy and often after a TURP, no fluid is released during orgasm.

Endorectal MRI: MRI study of the prostate that involves placing a probe into the rectum to better assess the prostate gland.

Enzyme: A chemical that is produced by living cells that causes chemical reactions to occur while not being changed itself.

EPCA, EPCA-2: An investigational prostate cancer marker that is plasma-based and appears to be highly specific for cancer.

Epidural anesthesia: A special type of anesthesia whereby pain medications are placed through a catheter in the back, into the fluid that surrounds the spinal cord.

Erectile dysfunction: The inability to achieve and/or maintain an erection satisfactory for the completion of sexual performance.

Estrogen: A female hormone.

Experimental: An untested or unproven treatment or approach to treatment.

External-beam radiation therapy: Use of radiation that passes through the skin and is focused for maximal effect on a target organ, such as the prostate, to kill cancer cells.

F

Food and Drug Administration (FDA): Agency responsible for the approval of prescription medications in the United States.

Fistula: An abnormal passage or communication, usually between 2 internal organs, or leading from an internal organ to the surface of the body.

Field effect: Widespread molecular changes in normal or relatively normal tissue that predispose a person to cancer.

Flare reaction: A temporary increase in tumor growth and symptoms that is caused by the initial use of LHRH agonists: It is prevented by the use of an antiandrogen 1 week before LHRH agonist therapy begins.

Fluoroscopy: Use of a fluoroscope, a radiologic device that is used for examining deep structures by means of X-rays.

Foley catheter: A latex or silicone catheter that drains urine from the bladder.

Free PSA: The PSA present that is not bound to proteins. It is often expressed as a ratio of free PSA to total PSA in terms of percent, which is the free PSA divided by the total PSA × 100.

Frequency: A term used to describe the need to urinate often.

Frozen section: A preliminary quick evaluation of tissue, removed a the time of biopsy or during surgery, by the pathologist who freezes the sample of tissue and shaves off a thin slice to examine under the microscope.

G

Gastrointestinal (GI): Related to the digestive system and/or the intestines.

General anesthesia: Anesthesia which involves total loss of consciousness.

Genetics: A field of medicine that studies heredity.

Genito-urinary tract: The urinary system (kidney, ureters and bladder, and urethra) and the genitalia (in the male the prostate, seminal vesicles, vas deferens, and testicles).

Gland: A structure or organ that produces substances that affect other areas of the body.

Gleason grade: A commonly used method to classify how cells appear in cancerous tissues; the less the cancerous cells look like normal cells, the more malignant the cancer; two numbers, each from 1 to 5, are assigned to the two most predominant types of cells present. These two numbers are added together to produce the Gleason score. Higher numbers indicate more aggressive cancers.

GnRH antagonist: A form of hormone therapy which works at the level of the brain to directly suppress the production of testosterone without initially raising the testosterone level.

Gracilis myoplasty: A surgical procedure whereby a muscle in the leg, the gracilis muscle, is repositioned around the urethra.

Gynecomastia: Enlargement or tenderness of the male breast(s).

H

Hematospermia: The presence of blood in the ejaculate (semen).

Hematuria: The presence of blood in the urine. It may be gross (visible) or microscopic (only detected under the microscope).

Hemibody: Half of the body.

Hereditary: Inherited from one's parents or earlier generations.

Heredity: The passage of characteristics from parents to their children by genes (genetic material).

Hernia: A weakening in the muscle that leads to a bulge, often in the groin.

Hesitancy: A delay in the start of the urine stream during voiding.

High grade: Very advanced cancer cells.

High intensity focused ultrasonography: A form of prostate cancer therapy that involves focusing high intensity ultrasound into the prostate to heat the prostate and destroy prostate cancer cells. It is being used in Europe but has not been approved in the United States.

High risk: More likely to have a complication or side effect.

Holistic: Considering man as a functioning whole or relating to the conception of man as a functioning whole.

Hormone refractory: Prostate cancer that is resistant to hormone therapy.

Hormone resistant: Prostate cancer that is resistant to hormone therapy.

Hormone therapy: The manipulation of the disease's natural history and symptoms through the use of hormones.

Hormones: Substances (estrogens and androgens) responsible for secondary sex characteristics (hair growth and voice change in men).

Hot flashes: The sudden feeling of being warm, may be associated with sweating and flushing of the skin, which occurs with hormone therapy.

Hyperplasia: Enlargement of an organ or tissue because of an increase in the number of cells in that organ or tissue, an example is benign prostatic hyperplasia.

Hyperthermia: Heating of the prostate to destroy tissue.

Hypoechoic: In ultrasonography, giving off few echoes; said of tissues or structures that reflect relatively few ultrasound waves directed at them.

Hypotension: Low blood pressure: May be associated with dizziness, fast heart rate and feeling weak and faint.

I

ICU (intensive care unit): A specialized area of the hospital where critically ill patients are taken care of.

IM: Intramuscular.

Immune response: The response of organs, tissues, blood cells, and substances that fight off infections, cancers, or foreign substances.

Immune system: A complex group of organs, tissues, blood cells and substances that work to fight off infections, cancers or foreign substances.

Impotence: See erectile dysfunction.

Incidental: Insignificant or irrelevant.

Incision: Cutting of the skin at the beginning of surgery.

Incontinence: Leakage of a substance without control: If the substance is urine, it is called urinary incontinence; if stool, it's called fecal incontinence. There are various kinds and degrees of urinary incontinence. Overflow incontinence is a condition in which the bladder retains urine after voiding, and as a result, urine leaks out, similar to a full cup under the faucet. Stress incontinence is the involuntary leakage of urine during periods of increased bladder pressure, such as coughing, laughing, and sneezing.

Total incontinence is the inability of the sphincter and urethra to prevent leakage of urine from the bladder.

Indications: The reasons for undertaking a specific treatment.

Infarct: An area of dead tissue resulting from a sudden loss of its blood supply.

Inflammation: Swelling, redness, pain, and irritation as the result of injury, infection, or surgery.

Informed consent: Permission given by a patient for a particular treatment after the patient has been notified of the indications for the procedure, the possible benefits and risks of the procedure, and alternative procedures that could be performed for the patient's condition.

Inpatient: A patient who is admitted to the hospital for treatment.

Integrative treatment: Treatments that are designed to work together.

Intermittency: An inability to complete voiding and empty the bladder with one single contraction of the bladder: A stopping and starting of the urine stream during urination.

Internist: A medical doctor who specializes in the nonsurgical treatment of disease and disease prevention.

Interstitial: Within an organ, such as interstitial brachytherapy, whereby radioactive seeds are placed into the prostate.

Intravenous: Into the veins.

Invasive: In cancer means the spread of the cancer beyond the site where it initially developed into surrounding tissues.

Investigator: A doctor or other individual who is involved with an experimental study or clinical trial.

IV: Intravenous.

IVP (intravenous pyelogram): A radiologic study, in which a contrast material (dye) is injected into the veins and is picked up by the kidneys and passed out into the urine, which allows one to visualize the urinary tract.

K

Kidney: One of a pair of organs that are responsible for eliminating chemicals and fluid from the body.

L

Laparoscopic radical prostatectomy: Removal of the entire prostate, seminal vesicles, and part of the vas deferens via the laparoscope.

Laparoscopy: Surgery performed through small incisions with visualization provided by a small fiberoptic instrument and fine instruments that fit through the small incisions.

Laser: A concentrated beam of high-energy light that is used in surgery.

LHRH analogue: A medication that tells the brain to tell the testicles to stop producing testosterone. It may initially raise serum testosterone, thus it is combined with an antiandrogen in men with metastatic prostate cancer.

LHRH antagonist: A medication that tells the brain to tell the testicles to stop producing testosterone. Not associated with an initial increase of testosterone.

Libido: Sex drive, interest in sex.

Lifestyle: The way a person chooses to live.

Lobe: A part of an organ: There are 5 distinct lobes in the prostate: 2 lateral lobes, 1 middle, an anterior, and a posterior.

Local anesthesia: Control of pain in a localized area of the body.

Local recurrence: The return of cancer to the area where it was first identified.

Localized: Confined, limited, contained to a specific area.

Low-grade: Cancer that does not appear aggressive, advanced.

Luteinizing hormone-releasing hormone (LHRH) analogues: A class of drugs that prevent testosterone production by the testes.

Lycopene: A substance found in tomatoes that has anticancer effects.

Lymph: A clear fluid that is found throughout the body: Lymph fluid helps fight infections.

Lymph node(s): Small bean-shaped glands that are found throughout the body: Lymph fluid passes through the lymph nodes, which filter out bacteria, cancer cells, and toxic chemicals.

Lymph node dissection: In the case of prostate cancer, pelvic lymph node dissection, which is the surgical removal of the lymph nodes in the pelvis to determine if prostate cancer has spread to the these nodes.

Lymphadenectomy: The technical term for lymph node dissection.

Lymphangiography: An X-ray test in which contrast is injected into the lymph vessels to determine if there is any blockage/tumor spread to the lymph nodes.

Lymphocele: A collection of lymph fluid in an area of the body.

M

Male sling: A procedure to promote urinary continence in which a piece of tissue is placed under the urethra to act as a hammock or buttress.

Malignancy: Uncontrolled growth of cells that can spread to other areas of the body and cause death.

Malignant: Cancerous, with the potential for uncontrolled growth and spread.

Medical oncologist: See oncologist.

Metastatic cancer: Cancer that has spread outside of the organ or structure in which it arose to another area of the body.

Metastatic recurrence: The return of cancer in an area of the body that is not the site where it originally developed.

Metastases: See Metastatic Cancer.

Microscopic: Small enough that a microscope is needed to see it.

Moderately differentiated: An intermediate grade of cancer as based on pathological evaluation of the tissue.

Molecular biology: The part of biology that deals with the formation, structure, and activity of macromolecules that are essential for life, such as nucleic acids.

Morbidity: Unhealthy results and complications resulting from treatment.

Mortality: Death related to disease or treatment.

MRI (magnetic resonance imaging): A study that is similar to a CT scan in that it allows one to see internal structures in detail, but it does not involve radiation.

Multifocal: Found in more than one area.

N

Natural treatment: Means derived from the earth, its plants, or animals: Natural doesn't always mean better for you.

Negative: A test result that does not show what one is looking for.

Neoadjuvant therapy: The use of a treatment, such as chemotherapy, hormone therapy, and radiation therapy, before surgery.

Neoplastic: Malignant, cancerous.

Nephrostomy tube: A tube that is placed through the back into the kidney and allows for drainage of urine from that kidney.

Nerve-sparing: With regard to prostate cancer, it is the attempt to not damage or remove the nerves that lie on either side of the prostate gland that are in part responsible for nor-

mal erections. Injury to the nerves can cause erectile dysfunction.

Nocturia: Awakening at night with the desire to void.

Noninvasive: Not requiring any incision or the insertion of an instrument or substance into the body.

Nucleic acids: Any of a group of complex compounds found in all living cells. Nucleic acids in the form of DNA and RNA control the functions of cells and heredity.

Nutrition: The science or study that deals with food and nourishment, especially in humans.

O

Obturator nerve: A nerve located in the pelvis near the pelvic lymph nodes that controls movement of the leg.

Occult cancer: Cancer that is not detectable through standard physical exams; symptom-free disease.

Oncologist: A medical specialist who is trained to evaluate and treat cancer.

Orchiectomy: Removal of the testicle(s).

Organ: Tissues in the body that work together to perform a specific function, e.g., the kidneys, bladder, heart.

Organ-confined disease: Prostate cancer that is apparently confined to the prostate clinically or pathologically; not going beyond the edges of the prostate capsule.

Osteoblastic lesion: Pertaining to plain X-ray of a bone, increased density of bone seen on X-ray when there is extensive new bone formation due to cancerous destruction of the bone.

Osteolytic lesion: Pertaining to plain X-ray of a bone, refers to decreased density of bone seen on X-ray when there is destruction and loss of bone by cancer.

Osteoporosis: The reduction in the amount of bone mass, leading to fractures after minimal trauma.

Overflow incontinence: The involuntary loss of urine related to incomplete emptying of the bladder.

P

PAP (prostatic acid phosphatase): A chemical that was once used to try to determine if the prostate cancer had spread outside of the prostate.

Palliative: Treatment designed to relieve a particular problem without necessarily solving it, e.g., palliative therapy is given in order to relieve symptoms and improve quality of life, but it does not cure the patient.

Palpable: Capable of being felt during a physical examination by an experienced doctor: In the case of prostate cancer, this refers to an abnormality of the prostate that can be felt during a rectal examination.

Partin tables: Tables that are developed based on results of the PSA, clinical stage, and Gleason score involving thousands of men with prostate cancer: These tables are used to predict the likelihood that prostate cancer has spread to the lymph nodes or seminal vesicles, penetrated the capsule, or remains confined to the prostate The tables were developed by Dr. Partin at Johns Hopkins University.

Pathologist: A doctor trained in the evaluation of tissues under the microscope to determine the presence/absence of disease.

Pelvic floor muscle exercises: Exercises that help one strengthen muscles that aid in the control of urinary incontinence.

Pelvis: The part of the body that is framed by the hip bones.

Penile clamp: A device placed around the penis to prevent urine leakage.

Penile prosthesis: A device that is surgically placed into the penis which allows an impotent individual to have an erection.

Penis: The male organ that is used for urination and intercourse.

Percutaneous: Through the skin.

Perineal: Refers to an incision made behind the scrotum and in front of the anus: The prostate can be removed through a perineal incision.

Perineal prostatectomy: Removal of the entire prostate, seminal vesicles, and part of the vas deferens through an incision made in the perineum.

Perineum: The area of the body that is behind the scrotum and in front of the anus.

Periprostatic: That tissue that lies immediately adjacent to the prostate.

Permanent section: The formal preparation of tissue removed at the time of surgery for microscopic evaluation.

Pharmacology: The science of drugs, including their composition, uses, and effects.

PIN (prostatic intraepithelial neoplasia): An abnormal area in a prostate biopsy specimen that is not cancerous, but may become cancerous or be associated with cancer elsewhere in the prostate.

Plasma: The liquid component of the blood.

Placebo: A fake medication ("candy pill") or treatment that has no effect on the body that is often used in experimental studies to determine if the experimental medication/treatment has an effect.

Ploidy status: The genetic status of cells, similar to the grade.

Pneumatic sequential stockings: Inflatable stockings that squeeze the legs intermittently to decrease the risk of a blood clot in the legs.

Poorly differentiated: High-grade, aggressive cancer as determined by microscopic evaluation of the tissue.

Positive biopsy: For cancer, it is the detection of cancer in the tissue.

Positive margin: The presence of cancer cells at the cut edge of tissue removed during surgery: A positive margin indicates that there may be cancer cells remaining in the body.

Posterior: The rear or back side.

Priapism: An erection that lasts longer than 4 to 6 hours.

Proctitis: Inflammation of the rectum.

Prognosis: The long-term outlook or prospect for survival and recovery from a disease.

Progression: The continued growth of cancer or disease.

Prostate: A gland that surrounds the urethra and is located just under the bladder: It produces fluid that is part of the ejaculate (semen) This fluid provides some nutrient to the sperm.

Prostate specific antigen (PSA):
A chemical produced by benign and cancerous prostate tissue: The level tends to be higher with prostate cancer.

Prostate surgery: Surgery for benign and malignant diseases of the prostate.

Prostatectomy: Any of several surgical prcedures in which part or all of the prostate gland is removed. These procedures include laparoscopic radical prostatectomy, radical perineal prostatectomy, radical retropubic prostatectomy, and transurethral prostatectomy (TURP).

ProstaScint: A specialized study that detects an antigen called the prostate-specific antigen: It is helpful in picking up recurrent prostate cancer.

Prostatitis: Inflammation or infection of the prostate gland.

Prosthesis: An artificial device used to replace the lost normal function of a structure or organ in the body.

Protocol: Research study used to evaluate a specific medication or treatment.

Proton-beam therapy: In conjunction with external-beam therapy, use of powerful beams of photons that are focused onto the prostate.

PSA density: The amount of PSA per gram of prostate tissue (PSA/g of prostate tissue).

PSA nadir: The lowest value that the PSA reaches during a particular treatment.

PSA progression: Increase in PSA after treatment of prostate cancer.

PSA velocity: The rate of change of the PSA over a period of time (change in PSA/change in time).

Q

QD: Daily

QID: Four times a day

QOD: Every other day

Quality of life: An evaluation of healthy status relative to the patient's age, expectations, and physical and mental capabilities.

R

Radiation oncologist: A physician who treats cancer through the use of radiation therapy.

Radiation proctitis: Inflammation of the rectal lining as a result of radiation therapy.

Radiation therapy: Use of radioactive beams or implants to kill cancer cells.

Radical perineal prostatectomy:
Removal of the entire prostate and seminal vesicles for prostate cancer through a perineal incision.

Radical retropubic prostatectomy: The surgical removal of the entire prostate plus the seminal vesicles and part of the vas deferens through an incision that extends down from the umbilicus (belly button).

Randomized: The process of assigning patients to different forms of treatment in a research study in a random manner.

Recurrence: The reappearance of disease: The recurrence may be clinical (a physical finding) or laboratory (e.g., a rise in the PSA).

Refractory: Resistant to therapy.

Regression: Reduction in the size of a single tumor or reduction in the number and/or size of several tumors.

Retention: Difficulty in emptying the bladder of urine, may be complete, in which one is unable to void, or partial, in which urine is left in the bladder after voiding.

Retropubic approach: See Radical retropubic prostatectomy.

Risk: The chance or probability that a particular event will or will not happen.

Robotic-assisted radical prostatectomy: A radical prostatectomy performed with the assistance of a robot.

S

Salvage: A procedure intended to "rescue" a patient after a failed prior therapy, e.g., a salvage radical prostatectomy after failed external-beam therapy.

Scrotum: The pouch of skin that contains the testicles.

Screening: Examination or testing of a group of individuals to separate those who are well from those who have an undiagnosed disease or defect or who are at high risk.

Semen: The whitish fluid that is released during ejaculation.

Seminal vesicles: Glandular structures that are located above and behind the prostate: They produce fluid that is part of the ejaculate.

Sensitivity: The probability that a diagnostic test can correctly identify the presence of a particular disease.

Side effect: A reaction to a medication or treatment.

Sign: Objective evidence of a disease, i.e., something that the doctor identifies.

Soy: Soy products are made from soy beans, a legume. Soy products are high in isoflavones, which may be helpful in preventing cancer cell growth.

Specificity: The probability that a diagnostic test can correctly identify the absence of disease.

Sphincter: A muscle that surrounds and by its tightening causes closure of an opening, e.g., the sphincter at the bladder outlet and in the urethra.

Stage: A term used to describe the size and the extent of a cancer.

Staging: The process of determining the extent of disease, which is helpful in determining the most appropriate treatment: Often involves physical examination, blood testing, and X-ray studies.

Stress incontinence: The involuntary loss of urine during sudden rises in intra-abdominal pressure, e.g., with coughing, laughing, sneezing, or picking up heavy objects.

Stricture: Scarring as a result of a procedure or an injury that causes narrowing and in the case of the urethra may constrict the flow of urine.

Supplement: Something that completes or is in addition: A medication/therapy that is used in addition to another medication/therapy.

Symptom: Subjective evidence of a disease, i.e., something a patient describes, e.g., pain in abdomen.

T

Taxane: A family of drugs that inhibits cell growth by stopping cell division.

Testis: One of two male reproductive organs that are located within the scrotum and produce testosterone and sperm.

Testosterone: The male hormone or androgen that is produced primarily by the testes and is needed for sexual function and fertility.

Three-dimensional (3-D) conformal radiation therapy: A variation of external-beam radiation therapy in which a computer, CT scan images, and a brace are used to focus the radiation more directly on the target organ/location.

TID: Three times a day.

Tissue: Specific type of material in the body, e.g., muscle, hair.

TNM System: The most common staging system for prostate cancer. It reflects the size of the tumor, nodal disease, and metastatic disease.

Total androgen blockade: The total blockage of all male hormones (those produced by the testicles and the adrenals) using surgery and/or medications.

Total PSA: The combination of bound and free PSA.

Transferrin: A chemical in the body that has been shown to stimulate the growth of prostate cancer.

Transperineal: Through the perineum.

Transrectal: Through the rectum.

Transurethral: Through the urethra.

Transurethral prostatectomy: See TURP.

Transrectal ultrasound: Visualization of the prostate by the use of an ultrasound probe placed into the rectum.

Tumor: Abnormal tissue growth that may be cancerous or noncancerous (benign).

Tumor markers: Chemicals that can be used to detect and follow the treatment of certain cancers.

Tumor volume: The amount of cancer present in an organ.

TURP (transurethral prostatectomy): A surgical technique performed under anesthesia using a specialized instrument similar to the cystoscope that allows the surgeon to remove the prostatic tissue that is bulging into the urethra and blocking the flow of urine through the urethra. After a TURP, the outer rim of the prostate remains.

U

Undergrading: A term that indicates that the grade of cancer is worse than that found in the biopsy tissue.

Understaging: The assignment of an overly low clinical stage at initial diagnosis because of the difficulty of assessing the available information with accuracy.

Ultrasound: A technique used to look at internal organs by measuring reflected sound waves.

Unit: Term referring to a pint of blood.

Ureters: Tubes that connect the kidneys to the bladder, through which urine passes into the bladder.

Urethra: The tube that runs from the bladder neck to the tip of the penis through which urine passes.

Urge incontinence: The involuntary loss of urine associated with the urge to urinate and is related to an overactive bladder.

Urgency: The feeling that one needs to urinate right away.

Urinary incontinence: The unintentional loss of urine.

Urinary retention: The inability to urinate leading to a filled bladder.

Urologist: A doctor that specializes in the evaluation and treatment of diseases of the genito-urinary tract in men and women.

V

Vas deferens: A tiny tube that connects the testicles to the urethra through which sperm passes.

Vasectomy: A procedure in which the vas deferens are cut and tied off, clipped, or cauterized to prevent the exit of sperm from the testicles: It makes a man sterile.

W

Watchful waiting: Active observation and regular monitoring of a patient without actual treatment.

Well-differentiated: A low-grade cancer as determined by microscopic analysis.

Whitmore-Jewett System: An alternative staging system for prostate cancer.

X

X-ray: A type of high-energy radiation that can be used at low levels to make images of the internal structures of the body and at high levels for radiation therapy.

Z

Zones: An area of the prostate distinguished from adjacent areas.

Index

Note: A *t* following a page number indicates a table; an italic page number indicates a figure.

Watchful waiting (*continued*)
    description of, 127–129
    hormone therapy and, 140
    pros of, 129
    rising PSA after radical prostatectomy
      and, 138
Weight gain, prostate cancer and, 14
White blood cell count, low, chemotherapy
    and, 69
White males, bone density and, 118

Whitmore-Jewett System of staging, 49–50
Wills, 172
Women, prostate-specific antigen and, 4

Y

Yang Proscheck, 9

Z

Zones, prostate gland, 3